THE
WONDER
OF THE
BRAIN

THE
WONDER
OF THE
BRAIN

GOPI KRISHNA

UBSPD
UBS Publishers' Distributors Ltd.
New Delhi • Bombay • Bangalore • Madras
Calcutta • Patna • Kanpur • London

UBS Publishers' Distributors Ltd.

5 Ansari Road, New Delhi-110 002
Phones: 3273601, 3266646 ☆ *Cable* : ALLBOOKS ☆ *Fax* : (91) 11-327-6593
e-mail: ubspd.del@smy.sprintrpg.ems.vsnl.net.in
Apeejay Chambers, 5 Wallace Street, Mumbai-400 001
Phones : 2076971, 2077700 ☆ *Cable* : UBSIPUB ☆ *Fax* : 2070827
10 First Main Road, Gandhi Nagar, Bangalore-560 009
Phones : 2263901, 2263902, 2253903 ☆ *Cable* : ALLBOOKS ☆ *Fax* : 2263904
6, Sivaganga Road, Nungambakkam, Chennai-600 034
Phone : 8276355 ☆ *Cable* : UBSIPUB ☆ *Fax* : 8270189
8/1-B, Chowringhee Lane, Calcutta-700 016
Phones : 2441821, 2442910, 2449473 ☆ *Cable* : UBSIPUBS ☆ *Fax* : 2450027
5 A, Rajendra Nagar, Patna-800 016
Phones : 652856, 653973, 656170 ☆ *Cable* : UBSPUB ☆ *Fax* : 656169
80, Noronha Road, Cantonment, Kanpur-208 004
Phones : 369124, 362665, 357488 ☆ *Fax* : 315122

Copyright © Gopi Krishna

Published in arrangement with
F.I.N.D. Research Trust
R.R. 5 Flesherton
Ontario, Canada
N0C 1E0

First Indian Reprint   1993
Second Indian Reprint 1994
Third Indian Reprint   1997

Printed at Replika Press (P) Ltd.
A-229, DSIDC Industrial Area, Narela, Delhi-110040

CONTENTS

By the Same Author

Kundalini, The Evolutionary Energy in Man
(An Autobiography)

The Biological Basis of Religion and Genius

The Secret of Yoga

Higher Consciousness

The Awakening of Kundalini

The Riddle of Consciousness

The Dawn of a New Science

Secrets of Kundalini in Panchastavi

Yoga, A Vision of Its Future

The Real Nature of Mystical Experience

Kundalini in Time and Space

The Shape of Events to Come

Reason and Revelation

The Present Crisis

The Way to Self-knowledge

From the Unseen

INTRODUCTION

Of all the mysteries that still remain to be solved by modern science, none is more intriguing, nor more important than the question of how the brain works. Despite the great strides made in the last few decades in learning how the brain is constituted and how it relates to perception, behaviour and cognition, the questions about what our consciousness really is and the exact role the brain plays in manifesting it, are still very much to be answered.

Science is based on the supposition that what we perceive with our brain, through the five senses, enhanced by recording and measuring instruments, is accurate, consistent and complete. Yet the results of the explorations of subatomic physics into the roots of matter have shown that this picture is far from complete. This is further emphasized by the enigmas posed by psychic phenomena, which seem to defy some of the laws of the physical world. These phenomena indicate that in certain individuals, the brain has rudimentary faculties of a different order than those of which we are aware and which we are only beginning to comprehend.

Even so, very little thought has been given to what changes would occur in our world-picture, and to the status of scientific knowledge, if the standard sensory input we all use were to be enhanced by the development of additional channels of perception in the brain.

In this book, Gopi Krishna describes what the nature of these evolving faculties are and how they will radically alter the current notions about consciousness and its place in our scheme of reality. He was uniquely qualified to do this because of the amazing transformation he underwent over a period of some forty-five years, beginning at the age of 34, when he awakened Kundalini. His description of this process, the subject of his autobiography, *Kundalini — The Evolutionary Energy in Man*, has become a classic in the literature of Yoga.

As the result of the heightening of his perceptive faculties, he concluded that the different mental states he experienced were the direct result of physical changes occurring at the subtlest levels of his brain and nervous/system. He was actually able to observe the flow of life-energy, or *prana*, throughout his body. Once the existence of the biological factors responsible for expanded consciousness, paranormal faculties and illumination are verified by science, he says, a revolution will occur in our basic understanding of what the physical world is and how consciousness relates to it.

                                                              Eileen Holland

1
Mystics — True and False

The true and the fake men of God have been living side by side in India for thousands of years. The ubiquitous hashish smoker often presents the same appearance and carries the same accoutrements as the genuine sadhu who wanders from place to place in search of truth. The former can be easily picked out, sitting cross-legged alone or in groups near holy shrines and places of pilgrimage, with matted hair and wiry bodies, besmeared with ashes, bloodshot eyes and gleaming teeth, blowing out clouds of smoke from their 'chilams' held in a characteristic way in their hands. The godmen of India are not all of the same class or rank. There are feudal lords, with large possessions and crowds of followers, their subjects among them. The highly learned and accomplished, as well as the ignorant and the raw, are found in their ranks.

The fear of the supernatural, the deep-rooted belief in the magical and the miraculous, as also the hunger for religious experiences, existing in countless human hearts, have provided, from the remotest periods of time, an honourable and congenial occupation for myriads, who choose piety and asceticism as a way of life. They are known as holymen, saints, sadhus, dervishes, faqirs and yogis and are met everywhere. There are millions in India, belonging to different orders and sects, distinguishable from each other by their dress, appearance, the state of hair, mark on the forehead, earrings and the equipment they carry when moving from place to place.

The majority of them consists of god-fearing, honest souls, driven to this mode of life by necessity, want, bereavement, discord with the family, misfortune, loss, distaste for the world, desire for escape, wanderlust, sloth, thirst for the supernatural or a deep-rooted urge for self-awareness and the Vision of God. What befalls them on the path, what kind of life they lead and what measure of success they achieve is hard to tell, for everyone of them, like everyone of us, the hero of his own drama of life, behind the impassive mask he presents to the world, experiences the same ups and downs, pleasures and pains, successes and failures, hopes and despairs, in his own self-chosen vocation, as we do in ours.

But, as in other walks of life, along with the sincere and the true there are also the clever and the artful, who do not scruple to use monasticism or the robes of an ascetic as stepping stones to affluence, honor and fame. Both types devote many years of their lives to preparing themselves for the role—a rather difficult one—demanding great intelligence, skill and tact to impress the seeking crowds, the shrewd and the gullible both. The former equip themselves for the part with a sincere desire to disseminate the knowledge they possess and teach others the disciplines they have themselves learned from their teachers, at great sacrifice, with an unshakable faith in their potency. The latter train themselves in or are naturally endowed with the art of play-acting and dissimulation to present a facade of holiness, supernatural prowess, divine intoxication and bubbling joy to the world. To a keen observer, the pose at once becomes obvious, but the simple and the credulous take many years, endure many trials and undergo heavy costs to come to the same conclusion.

The few who take to tartuffery spend years in the study of scriptures and literature on Yoga or the occult, practice postures of the body, attain proficiency in meditation and learn to bring about semi-conscious trance conditions at will by autohypnosis or highly diminished breathing or drugs. They sometimes add to these accomplishments, sleight-of-hand, sophistry and a handy store of metaphysical cant picked up from the Vedanta or other systems of philosophy in India. Thus equipped with a studiously cultivated pose, gestures, expression of the eyes, a constantly playing smile on the lips, simulated ecstacy, sometimes with the whites of the eyes turned upward, they become a powerful center of attraction, counting their followers and disciples in hundreds and thousands everywhere.

The paradoxical element in human nature or their own altruistic tendencies impels some of them to devote themselves to acts of charity, compassion, benevolence and other wholesome pursuits, believing sincerely in the axiom that the end justifies the means. But there also are some who pose as saints, ascetics, or yogis with purely selfish or mercenary aims. Surrounded by their devotees, disciples and camp-followers, they present an imposing spectacle which the media, always in search of the spectacular, the bizarre and the uncommon, carry round the world, helping unwittingly in attracting more and more spectators and dupes to the show. They are not to blame, as dissimulation and disguise are hard to detect under the outer dress of sanctity and saintliness.

The ones with the gift of gab, a facile pen or skill at repartee become instant successes. There is a magic in the territory of the supernatural, which attracts the lover of the occult, the credulous and the superstitious, as a flame attracts a moth. Try as one might, one cannot dissuade a believer from lending credence to palpable fiction or in relying on the efficacy of methods, formulas or spells, absurd and irrational on the face of them. The same is true of numerous widely read books purporting to impart knowledge of the occult, which are packed with nothing but supernatural fiction and made-up stories of thrilling adventures and bizarre encounters with yogis, lamas, adepts, magicians and the rest in a far-off land where these rare beings abound. The more incredible and fantastic the tale, the more is the fascination exercised by it on the occult fans. What the readers probably seek is not the truth but the excitement of these bizarre accounts and ghostly narratives. No wonder some of them become best-sellers and are eagerly sought for.

At this point another magic begins to operate. Some even among the learned, from whom one would expect a sober and critical assessment of the phantasmagoria presented in the books, not to be left behind, nod their approval and jump on the band-wagon, until the spell is broken and the story is seen in its real color, a figment of the authors brain used opportunely in a clever bid for fortune. It is incredible that, after so many debacles witnessed in recent years—for instance the exposure of psychic tricksters, the disillusionment with mind-culture techniques, the waning popularity of godmen and miracle-yogis, the havoc caused by the drug experiment, the blank drawn in the search for Siddhas and Masters, the horrors of cultism and the exploded myths of occult anecdotes—there should not be even the shadow of an attempt to stop this illicit commerce and save millions of people from the grip of vendors of the supernatural, as unscrupulous and greedy as those in any other sphere of human interest. The stir caused by the newspaper reports of the shocking malpractice in this holy trade is usually followed by an unbroken lull, until the calm is broken by other shattering news of the same kind, to be followed by silence once again.

The real saint and the professional godman are poles apart. The yogi, dextrous in asanas, ready to suspend his breathing or to arrest his pulse or to endure burial underground for days, might be no better than the mendicant who reclines on a bed of sharp nails or hangs head down from a tree, over a pungently smoking fire, for a living. Large numbers of them are only rare objects of curiosity for their uncanny contortions, mastery over vital functions or immunity to pain; but when it comes to knowledge of the super-mundane are often as ignorant, if not even more, than those who crowd around them in wonder at their extraordinary feats. The famous mystic-poetess, Lalleshwari, with her usual brevity of expression, has portrayed thus the agony of the mystical mind at the inability of the masses to distinguish a true ecstatic from the pretender and the sham:

> "Hard it is for a (limpid) pool of spring-water to be sighted in a maze of running streams, among which it is lost to the eye,
>
> Hard it is for a Royal Swan (a fabulous bird which can separate milk from water) to be noticed in a flock of crows,
>
> Hard it is for a man of learning to be known in a habitation of the ignorant,
>
> And hard it is for a man of God to be recognized in a den of thieves."

Commenting on the apathy of the multitudes towards the sublime state of self-awareness, Lalla sings:

> "How can a kite (which feeds on carrion) be appreciative of the taste of a falcon which eats only freshly killed prey?
>
> And can a barren woman know the intensity of the love of a mother for her child?
>
> How can a (smoking) torch perceive the beauty and mellowness of the light of a lamp?
>
> And how can a fly (fond of filth) understand the passion of a moth which burns itself over a flame?"

Of her own ordeals in facing the opprobrium of the uninformed crowd, she says:

> "Upon my forehead did I receive the abuse and the scorn of the world,
>
> And watched, unperturbed, calumny spreading in the front and the rear of me,
>
> Lalla I remained, steadfast in my love of God,
>
> Until I reached the 'Abode of Light'."

Guru Nanak, the founder of the Sikh faith and one of the greatest among the luminaries of India, exposes thus the false Yogi:

> "Yoga is neither in the patched coat, nor in the Yogi's staff,

nor in smearing oneself with ashes. Nor in wearing earrings, nor close-cropping the head, nor in blowing the horn. If one remaineth detached in the midst of attachments, one attaineth to the (true) state of Yoga. One becometh not a Yogi by mere talk. If one looketh upon all creation alike, one is acclaimed as a true Yogi. Yoga is not in abiding at the tombs or the crematoriums, nor in entering into pseudo-trance, Yoga consists not in roaming the world, nor in bathing in places of pilgrimage. If one remaineth detached in the midst of attachments, then, verily, one attaineth to the (true) state of Yoga.*"

There is something inhuman in the apathy shown by the people in general, scholars and laity alike, in understanding the real significance of Mystical Vision, in evoking a picture, however hazy it might be, of that sublime state, and in assessing its paramount importance for the race. There is something bizarre, I repeat, in the crass ignorance existing at present about the colossal dimensions of this experience and the conclusion that can be drawn from it, namely that the normal human mind is a prison for the soul, and that nature has already provided the key to open it to allow individuals to soar to freedom in regions of unspeakable glory and joy.

Why extreme asceticism, self-denial, retreat from the world, self-inflicted pain, self-imposed poverty or suppression of basic appetites have been a common practice for the travellers on this path is explained by the reason that the nature of the urge is not known nor has any serious attempt been made to understand its working so far. As in other spheres of human life, patient, painstaking and prolonged study were necessary to make this achievement easy and smooth. But, unfortunately, due to the mistaken notion that here the pilgrims travel in God's own territory, where magic, miracles and windfalls abound, where eccentric and irrational behaviour are the rule, suppression and

---

* Gopal Singh, *Guru Nanak*

denial of natural appetites the key to success, perverted thinking and aversion to the world the normal course of life, those who traversed the path, except for a few, seldom achieved success in this pious undertaking. Even where success was achieved, it was more often than not partial, attended by shadowy delusions, obsessions and eccentricities which have been as marked a feature of religious genius as of its secular counterpart.

It never took very long for recognition to come to men and women of extraordinary talent or doubts to linger on about their stature and worth. Even when forced to dwell in obscurity for awhile, the light they shed spread out at last. The brilliant galaxy of the highest genius in every branch of knowledge and skill is well before the eyes of most of the well-educated and well-informed people everywhere. Their identity is so well established and the productions so well known that no chance is left for an imitator or impersonator to pretend that he or she is one of them. Anyone who attempts such a foolish deception can never hope to escape instant detection and exposure at the hands of the outraged intelligentsia. In fact, it is inconceivable that even the most reckless and daring would ever attempt to impose on the credulity of the public in this case. The only exception can be the deluded and the disoriented, and it is well known that they sometimes do claim they are possessed by or in communication with the spirit of a distinguished scion of this family or even a reincarnation of one of them.

It is extremely unlikely that any sensible person would publicly dare to place himself in the same rank with a Plato or a Patanjali, a Kali-Dass or a Kant, a Galileo or a Mozart, a Rembrandt or a Hafiz, a Gandhi or an Emerson, without bringing upon himself the condemnation and the obloquy of the world. How does it happen then that in the still more exclusive province of the Divine everyone is allowed to wear whatever badge of honor he likes, to rank himself with whomsoever of high distinction he prefers without anybody lifting his little finger to contradict or condemn him?

It is a sad commentary on the mental acumen of this rational age that even those who claim to be the Lord God Himself or His Incarnation, or declare their parity with the Most High, thus out-ranking the greatest among the illuminati of the past, more widely known and honored than the highest among the secular geniuses, are taken at their word, to become the spiritual guides and preceptors of countless men and women until the light of publicity is turned off and they sink into the oblivion from which, all of a sudden, they had emerged.

Can anyone provide an answer to the paradox why, in this age of reason, when every event of history, every thought and motive behind human behaviour and every phenomenon of Nature has been subjected to the closest scrutiny and analysis with the result that even the innermost urges of human beings, the movements of the remotest stars, the configurations of distant planets, the topography of the ocean beds and the happenings in the very womb of earth stand explained, the learned should be so ill-informed about the extraordinary endowment that produced a towering genius like Moses, Buddha, Vasishtha, Vyasa, Socrates, Christ, Mohammed, Nanak and other great luminaries of the earth? What an irony of fate that the well-informed of today should be so ignorant about a phenomenon that was clearly known and recognized in Egypt and India, more than three thousand years before the birth of Christ, repeated since then time after time, with a shattering effect on society, at times, during the whole course of history to this day.

Can it be possible that the inane picture of the inner state of a mystic painted by some contemporary writers, with lights, sounds, fanciful or phantasmic visionary experiences, reminding one of hypnagogic or drug states, could have inspired a Buddha, a Christ, a Lao-Tse, a Shankaracharya, a Saint Paul or a Kabir or other great prophets and mystics of mankind to the sublime ideals they preached, the sacrifices they made or the exemplary lives they led. The mind's antipodes of Huxley and its fantastic dwellers are as far away from the lucidity experienced in the ecstatic trance as the shadows of night are from the clarity of day. We are making the same error about the transcendental plane as the scholars before the time of Copernicus did in respect of the universe perceptible to our physical senses. They allotted to the earth a position exactly the reverse of what it is in relation to the sun. Many of the current notions about mystical ecstasy are almost equally distant from the truth.

This doubt and confusion about the real nature of Mystical Vision and the mental endowment peculiar to the illuminati are prevalent not only today but have been so from remote periods of time. There are scores of ancient books on Yoga, Zen, Taoism and other spiritual disciplines in Sanskrit, Chinese, Japanese, Tibetan, Persian, Arabic and other languages, accepted as authoritative today, which clearly betray the ignorance of the authors about the real experience and show them as professionals or initiates of some order who, facile of pen, wrote down their treatises from book lore or oral tradition or from the teachings and sermons of their spiritual preceptors, without actual knowledge of the grand finale of the quest. I know how hard it is to convince the world of the truth of what I assert, and how necessary it is to provide external proof of the incredible change within. I, too, on my part, am as keen to furnish this testimony in support of the great secret it is my purpose to unveil.

The ego and vanity in man often stand in the way of his acceptance of the position that super-ordinary consciousness, to which he is a total stranger, can be possible for some members of the species to which he belongs. This frame of mind is often more pronounced in scholars who fondly believe that more and more extensive knowledge of the world and its infinitely varied phenomena, provided by poring over vast libraries of books, is the only expansion and advancement possible to the human mind. It cannot but be repugnant to a polymath to be told that there is a learning beyond his grasp, that the very nature of the mind can change and can soar to normally supersensible planes of being, which are inaccessible to the keenest intellect, however well informed and penetrating it might be.

We know that a child prodigy can work out enormous sums with lightning speed, impossible for the most expert mathematician, or excel acknowledged masters in music, chess, poetry or art. Do the present notions about mystical ecstasy or, the so-called 'peak experience' current among scholars, explain this phenomenon? Do the psychological explanations they offer for mystical experience or the self-drawn picture they have of it apply to genius also? If not, they are on the wrong track. The phenomenon of ecstasy is ten times more complex than what they assume it to be.

Whenever a great spiritual prodigy arose in India, the first ordeal before him was to convince the rank and file of his contemporaries of his extraordinary achievement. The life-stories of Buddha, Shankaracharya, Guru Nanak, and the recorded dialogues between the great sages of the Upanishads and the often well-placed and well-informed seekers who sought their guidance bear testimony to this fact. In the Bhagavad Gita, too, Arjuna puts the same question to Krishna in reply to the latter's comment that one only attains to Yoga when his intellect, bewildered by the scriptures, stands steady in Samadhi. For the present-day seeker, we can say 'bewildered by the welter of views expressed by the writers on the subject.'

Arjuna words his query thus: "What is the mark of him who is stable of mind, steadfast in Samadhi (Mystical Vision), Oh Keshava? How doth the stable-minded talk, how doth he sit, how walk?"

Krishna answers this pertinent question in the same way as an illuminati would answer it today: "When a man abandoneth, Oh Partha, all the desires of the heart and is satisfied in the Self by the Self" he says, "then he is called stable in mind." The words "satisfied in the Self by the Self" are significant. The reference is to the fascinating, blissful and highly gratifying inner world, now opened to the third eye of the adept—a world so exhilarating and transporting that the raptures and delights of the world of senses appear insignificant in comparison. This total satisfaction and joy, experienced at the discovery of the surpassing nature of one's own Self, is one of the most distinctive features of the ecstatic trance.

"He whose mind is free from anxiety amid pain," continues Krishna, "indifferent amid pleasures, loosened from passion, fear and anger, is called a sage of stable mind." Explaining these qualifications further, he says, "He who on every side is without attachments, whatever hap of fair or foul, who neither likes nor dislikes—of such a one the understanding is well-poised.... When again a tortoise draws in on all sides its limbs, he withdraws his senses from the objects of sense, then is his understanding well-poised."

Krishna gives another significant hint to Arjuna in the next verse. "The objects of sense, but not the relish for them," he says, "turn away from an abstemious dweller in the body and even relish turneth away from him after the Supreme is seen." In other words, the marvellous spectacle unfolded to the illuminated is so saturated with all that is beautiful, pure, harmonious and delightful in human experience that the mind turns away from the allurements and the pleasures of the earth.*

The inspired authors of the Bhagavad Gita, the Upanishads, Yoga Vasishtha, Dhammapada, the Bible, the Quran, the Adigranth, the Cloud of Unknowing, the Mathnavi and other masterpieces of spiritual literature have been as far above the ordinary run of pandits, yogis, sadhus, lamas, dervishes, fakirs, ascetics and saints as Homer, Dante, Kali-Das, Shakespeare and Goethe are above the common class of poets and scholars, however prolific or erudite they might have been. Spiritual genius is the most precious ornament to which the human mind can aspire. Its secret is still unknown. Its influence on societies has been the most powerful of all and is still unmatched by any other class of human beings. The tragedy has been that the stereotyped picture, drawn by many of the contemporary writers on Yoga, and its practices and postures, relatively unfamiliar to the West, has tended to create a wrong impression, that the ecstasy of western mystics and the Samadhi of Yogis are two dissimilar states of

---

* *Bhagavad-Gita,* Second Discourse, verses 55-59

spiritual perception. They are not. The genuine state is one and the same for Christians, Muslims, Hindus, Buddhists and Jews. There is no Christian Mysticism, Jewish Mysticism, Sufi Mysticism, Hindu Mysticism or Buddhist Mysticism. These arbitrary divisions are the creations of scholars, unfamiliar with the real experience. It has almost the same basic characteristics of all, and the same organic mechanism comes into operation in its manifestation. Variations occur where the experience is purely psychological, partaking of a delusory or dream-like character, which varies from person to person and, relatively speaking, leaves no lasting imprint on the personality of the subject.

Can there be any doubt about the position that, during the last twenty-five centuries, Buddha, Christ or Mohammed have been the most honored, most idolized, adored, discussed and talked about figures in history? The erudite who made them the objects of their studies, whether laudatory or critical, are nowhere seen in the resplendence which surrounds them. Even the greatest among secular geniuses emit only a feeble glow compared to the brightness of their splendor. The most scholarly volumes ever written make a poor show beside the popularity of the Bible, the Quran, the Bhagavad Gita or the Discourses of Buddha. What is the reason for this singularity? Why do the personalities and the utterances of the enlightened hold such a permanent place in and command such lasting devotion from the human heart? There must be a reason for it.

The argument that this idolization and homage do not emanate from the disciplined minds of scholars but from the superstitious fears of the commoners does not change the position, as it is hard to decide which of the two is right—the spontaneous acclaim and the instinctive homage of the majority or the cultivated cynicism of the learned few? Secondly, the scholars themselves depend for their own distinguished rank and position of authority on the same spontaneous approval and the instinctive recognition of their worth by the crowd.

I am constrained to say that ignorance of the nature of Mystical Experience is at the bottom of the confusion existing at present about Samadhi, the ultimate state of Yoga, or the mystical trance. There is no comparison at all between this surpassing state of lucidity and the so-called altered states of consciousness brought about by auto-suggestion, drugs, hypnosis or other artificial methods, which tamper with the normal functioning of the brain. Samadhi is as natural a state of consciousness as normal human awareness, with this important difference that, in the former, the relationship between the 'Knower' and the 'Known' is altered—the former assuming the proportions of an ocean in which the latter appears as an enchanted island, with activity and bustle, name and form, time and space, bound by cause and effect, and regulated by law—a perceptible and palpable creation in the midst of an Eternal Infinity of Being, experienced both within and without, but utterly mysterious and unfathomable to the last.

For ages the true servant of God and his pretentious rival have been rubbing shoulders with one another, almost indistinguishable in the fervor of the milling crowds around them, who could hardly perceive the yawning gulf of difference between the two. It could be that the modest contemplative, honest, unostentatious, simple and frugal, indifferent to worldly applause, pomp and show, might have even lost the palm to his clever impersonator, with abundant resources at his disposal, deeply learned in the scriptural lore, living in a royal state, lavish in charity and gifts— doled out with a purpose—surrounded by a bowing and fawning crowd of devotees and beneficiaries of his munificence, presenting to the world a silhouette of a richly blessed and miraculously endowed man of God.

How often had a true gently saint to watch patiently his own eclipse by a pretender or to endure dishonor and ridicule from the misled or incited public or the fanatical followers of a grandiloquent charlatan, rich with the offerings of the deceived votaries, forward, brazen and loud, it should not be hard to imagine. It is hard to distinguish between the two as there is no awareness of the fact that religion is the outcome of a deep-seated impulse in human beings, so powerful that at times it even outsizes the all-important reproductive urge. The result is that the

territory of faith has remained undemarcated and unwalled, to
serve as a haunt for the adventurer, side by side with the true
savant, as was the case with the province of healing and even of
other sciences in the past.

This is but one side of the picture. On the other, the rarely
found self-realized man of God has always been overwhelmingly
out-numbered by the fanatical anchorite, self-denying and self-
torturing, living on a handful of grain or a glass of milk, his naked
body covered with ashes or dressed in rags, silent and taciturn,
mumbling answers to enquiries; his appearance, gestures, posture,
habits and behaviour all calculated to convey the impression of
extreme piety, detachment from the world and immersion in the
silent ocean of the Self. Drawn by his weird appearance, extreme
penance, quaint answers to queries, gleaming, hypnotic eyes or
some other oddity, or a deliberately spread reputation for
miraculous powers, crowds surge around him, hopeful of a boon
or solution to a problem, only to waste years of life in search of
windfalls or treasure-troves which never become a reality.

Britain did not produce another Shakespeare, nor Germany
another Goethe, nor Greece Plato, nor China Confucius, nor
Persia Omar Khayyam, nor India Tulsi Dass, nor are they likely to
produce others of their stature for a long time to come. Like the
great secular geniuses, whose names are household words and
whose contributions to literature, art, philosophy and science
stand and might continue to stand unrivalled for centuries, there
have been spiritual geniuses in many lands, even rarer than the
former, whose achievements, too, will remain unmatched for
long. The tragedy is that many of us confuse this galaxy of stars of
the first magnitude with street performers and base our conclusions, not on the writings of Shakespeare himself, but on the
utterances of a minor actor in one of the magnificent dramas
authored by him.

This confusion about a historical reality and the present
apathy towards what I am unfolding will not last long, nor detract
from the value of the information given out, with meticulous
precision, as carefully sorted out and weighed as the data of an

experiment done in a laboratory. Nature does not keep her secrets forever. She has herself provided man with the equipment to ferret them out. Others will rise to support and supplement what I say. The experience is so extraordinary that it is easy to disbelieve it amid the hard realities of mundane life. Only they whose eyes are opened to this glory, biding unnoticed in the interior of every human being, can understand the difference between this hard-to-reach fount of happiness and the evanescent joy found in the pursuit of wealth, position or distinction which, at the end, turns out to have been the chase of a will-o'-the-wisp, that we did not possess the acumen to detect at first.

There are strange notions current about godmen and saints not only in India, but also in other parts of the world. The teachings of religion, the stories and legends current about the austerities performed and the miracles wrought by holy men of yore, belief in the supernatural, inherent in countless minds, and the prevalent ideas about the heavenly reward, awaiting the saintly and the pious have all tended to paint an inaccurate picture of the enlightened class. Many people, when visiting a saint, try to find in his appearance, facial expression, the look of the eyes, gestures or talk some hint or feature corresponding to the image already present in their mind. Where no such indication exists, their imagination, fastening on some peculiarity in the visage or the pose, interprets it as the distinctive mark which they seek. Lured by their own fancy, they surrender their own will to another as a slave does to his master, hovering round their idol, till the charm is broken by accident, and they find that the object of their veneration is no more hierarchic than they are.

The notion that one who has attained to sainthood must possess miraculous powers is common. The religious-minded and the pious are more prone to this idea. He must have something to distinguish him from the average class of human beings. His chastity, austerities and penances must have won some super-earthly prize, which is denied to others. His daily meditation and spiritual exercises must have brought to him the control of the occult forces of nature and opened his eyes to secrets which are veiled from everyone else. The crowds that throng the ashrams or apartments of holymen and saints mostly consist of those who believe in their sanctity and super-human stature. I am not surprised, therefore, when some of my visitors and correspondents expect a miracle from me either in solving a knotty problem or in bringing success to their spiritual quest.

Once when in West Germany, I was invited to meet a well-known psychiatrist. Accompanied by a friend, I went to his apartment in the afternoon. When we were seated, a friend of my host put a pack of cards in front of me on the table. The intention was that I should guess the cards to establish the truth of my profession, that I had won to mystical consciousness. I looked at the table and the cards in silence. The friend with me whispered in the ear of the gentleman that they had mistaken the purpose for which I had come, and that I had never pretended to psychic powers. The experience had a profound effect on my mind. It made me acutely aware of the fact that the 'mystic' was a stranger even to the learned. The world had a quaint picture of him, sometimes the very reverse of what it is in reality.

This frame of mind is based on a fundamental error, which treats mystical vision as a leap from the human state to the divine. The assumption is that one who has won access to the tran-scendental planes of creation must have gained supernatural powers also. This view is not consistent with the experience of the past. Miracles did not occur when man rose from the primate to the human state, nor when he gave up residence in caves to dwell in thatched huts or later in stately buildings in cities and towns.

No one entertains the idea that a saint loses his human appearance or his human habits of eating, drinking or sleeping. He might eat only a few grains of rice or drink only a draught of water every day, but he eats and drinks like others. He might sleep only an hour every night or after several nights, but he does sleep like other human beings. He might be lean or emaciated, well-built or obese, but he does look like the rest of us. It is admitted that he can be ill, grow aged and white-haired, pass away young or at a ripe age, but he does die and not live forever in the mortal frame. His body might rise from the grave or disappear from under the shroud or remain undecomposed for days, or only a few flowers might be left in the coffin in place of the corpse, or there might be a glow on his face or light radiate from his eyes at the end, but like all of us, his mortal coil does cease to exist one day.

It is thus clear that so far as his corporeal frame is concerned, the saint conforms to the pattern, with modifications here and there, which is common for all human beings. But when it comes to the mind, there is a phenomenal change which makes the others look like ants before him. He becomes a super-human colossus, with command over the elements and forces of nature and power of life and death or evil and good fortune over human beings. He can make torrential rain to stop, the sun to stand still, the earth to shake, the tempestuous ocean to be calm, the storm to subside, the river to roll back to allow him to pass, the dead to rise from their graves, severed heads to rejoin lifeless trunks, whole armies to retreat in disorder, mighty kings to tremble with fear, a handful of rice to appease the hunger of hundreds and do other miracles of this kind.

What is the reason for this diametrically opposite view concerning the limitations of the body and the unlimited powers of the mind in a man of God which even prevails today? The reason is that prophethood and saintliness have not been correctly understood so far, either in their biological content or in their psychology. The views current and even the scholarly disser-tations written are based on suppositions, legends, uncertain historical data or, sometimes, even the highly colored or fanciful self-revelations of mystics themselves. Confusion prevails because no critical physical or psychological study of a living mystic has been done so far. In fact, there is confusion about the distinctive characteristics of the mystic himself. Whatever is said or written is based on an imaginary picture of the entity, which varies from person to person, waiting for the day when the phenomenon is investigated on a living specimen and the results made known to the world.

The reasons why, as compared to the other branches of

knowledge, the real religious experience has remained an
unexplored province so far is because it failed to excite the same
interest and to command the same attention from the learned
during recent times as it had done in the past. Secondly, the
phenomenon has been so much shrouded in secrecy, superstition
and myth, and there are such fantastic tales current about the great
luminaries of spiritual knowledge that the impression gained by
an analytical mind is of folklore and legend rather than that of real
occurrences. In some cases, the accounts of some of the masters
themselves are too fantastic to be taken at their face value.
Another reason is that when, critically analyzed in the context of
the present-day knowledge of the Cosmos, the experience, as
interpreted by some of the mystics themselves, seems to be out of
all proportion to the puny stature of man and the giddy heights
which they believe they had attained.

The ancient Greek physician, Galen, is said to have left a
legacy of nearly five hundred treatises written on the art of healing,
out of which eighty are still extant. For centuries his position in
Greece, Rome and Arabia, in the world of medicine, was supreme.
He was the first to give a name to 'nerves' and to describe the
appearance of a cancerous tumour. During the middle ages, and
even later, he was considered an authority on pulse. But it cannot
be expected that his four score treatises would compare with the
works on therapy in our day. There would be many inaccuracies,
deficiencies and fanciful colorings about the causes and the
treatment of various diseases, as compared to the material
contained in the standard treatises of our time. Similarly, it is idle
to expect that the accounts of their experiences rendered by
medieval or ancient mystics would conform to our present-day
picture of what an accurate narrative should be.

We come across the same mixture of sound and useful
material mingled with what is inaccurate, fanciful and fictitious in
the books on alchemy, astrology, history, geography or natural
science, written in ancient times, in any part of the world. The
error has been that in the study on mystical literature, we rely
entirely on the accounts of the mystics, or their biographers or of

the other earlier writers on the subject, without having any guidelines or a model to judge which part of the accounts is correct, which exaggerated, which fictitious and which is a mixture of all of these ingredients put together. The learned have made the confusion more confounded by making this still obscure subject a venue for the exhibition of their own erudition by an extravagant use of pedantic phrases and terms which are as inappropriate to this sublime state of awareness as the language used in the books on pathology would be for wording the Gita or 'The Sermon on the Mount'.

There is no way to reach to the bottom of truth in this case, for the reason that highest sanctity is attached by the pious and the devout to these accounts, especially those in the sacred books of various faiths, which, for the believers, are sacrosanct. One, not credited with a stature as high as, or even higher than, that of the narrators of the experience, would not even be listened to, what to say of believed, if he has the audacity to find fault with them. The only way open is to repeat the experiments, under the supervision of teams of investigators, and to draw conclusions from it. The idea is not as impracticable as might be supposed. There are myriads of highly evolved human beings, especially among the talented class, who are mature for this experience. It can, therefore, be asserted with confidence that, even if the experiment is not done, there are bound to appear, at a not too distant date, spontaneous cases of illumination which will bear out what I say.

If the conclusion drawn by me, from my own experience, that the human brain is still in a state of organic evolution is correct, cases of spontaneous illumination, more so those maturing at an early age, are likely to increase in incidence in the years to come. Any well-informed man or woman of today, when face to face with the transcendental world, will not fail to recognize the landmarks I am pointing out, and to put the learned on the right track to what will be the zenith of human knowledge and achievement for ages to come. For this reason, I am not in the least disturbed when what I say passes unheeded in a world that has still to reconcile itself to the idea that true mystical vision represents the culmination of a long process of evolutionary changes in the subtle levels of the brain, as natural and as inevitable as the growth of an individual from childhood to maturity. The time may soon come when the rising generations, under the pressure of the growing urge for self-awareness, would not brook delay or trifling with an issue on which their happiness and peace of mind depends and take the initiative to rescue it from the present state of ambiguity or uncertainty and clear it of the dross that now sticks to it.

2
The Brain—
Forgotten Wizard

There is a serious gap in the knowledge of the learned about the working of the nervous system and the brain. They have no clear idea yet about the relationship between the neurons of the brain and the processes of thought, nor about the energy that fuels the former. It is surprising that, with such a void in our knowledge, relating to consciousness, any open-minded student can be so rigid in his views and dogmatic in his beliefs as is the case with not a few psychologists and biologists of our day.

It has been repeatedly asserted in my works, based not only on my experience of now more than forty years, but also on the experience of thousands of Yogis in India, Sufis in the Middle East, Western mystics and Taoists in China, that either as the result of appropriate disciplines or as a natural endowment, the activity of the reproductive system is reversible and that high-grade genius and every form of genuine mystical ecstasy result from the impact of this highly concentrated vital energy on the brain. Many of the present-day authorities on consciousness disbelieve this statement, because they see no conduit connecting the reproductive organ directly with the brain, nor is any such linkage mentioned in the present-day books on physiology.

Confident of their own erudition but, at the same time, oblivi-
ous to the lacunae in their knowledge, they reject and ridicule
what I say, not because they are wiser, but because they are not
able to see the error in their own thinking, based on a study of
which the bottom is missing. How can anyone contradict what I
say, when he does not even know the most rudimentary facts
about thought, namely how it is generated and in the process of
thinking, what energy do we consume? That the brain is nourished
by blood and sugar in the blood does not explain the position. If
thought has no substance, no material composition and is only an
incorporeal, etheric stuff, a living vacuum or thinking emptiness,
it cannot be nourished by blood; for that would involve transformation of matter into 'nothingness'—a predicament for science.
If it has substance, however subtle that might be, it must have an
energy system of its own to generate, replenish and renew it.
Where is that?

It is obvious that the materialists on the one hand and the
idealists on the other, the skeptics on this side and the believers
on that, the evolutionists and the creationists and all other mutually
contending schools of thought on this subject are wrangling over
an issue which, at the base, is paradoxical. No one of the contes-
tants knows, with certitude, what he is talking about. What is the
nature of the entity which forms the ground for the debate; what
is its relationship to the brain and its position in the universe?
Both sides deploy vast arrays of proofs, arguments and authorities
—all hypothetical—for no one knows positively anything basic
about the chief actor involved, namely the mind, save that it
exists.

One side takes it for granted that the world we see around is an
objective reality, and that the human mind is an accurately reflecting mirror which presents its true image before us. Everyone
believes that from whatever part of the earth we look at the
Universe, the picture would be the same. Even the latest concepts
of physics about the indeterminate nature of matter, at its ultra-
microscopic levels, do not change the position that our mind is an
accurate, unalterable and undoubtable instrument to observe,

assess and measure that which it perceives. All our present-day knowledge of science and philosophy is based on this assumption. All our ideas and beliefs are grounded on this supposition. Even our concepts of Soul, God and the Hereafter are the harvest of our faith in the integrity of our mind and the credibility of the intellect. To cast doubts on the reliability of the mind is to lose faith in the accuracy of our own observations and to create anarchy in every branch of human thought.

Time after time, the special class of men and women, known as mystics, visionaries and sages, tried to convince the crowds of a new form of perception attained by them, in which the objective Universe loses its corporeality and multiplicity to fuse into one indescribable and incomprehensible unity that bears no resemblance to the objective realities perceived before. As is natural, under the firm conviction that the normal human mind is the only accurate and standard instrument of cognition available to us, the experiences of this exclusive class are treated either as purely visionary excursions into the subliminal areas of consciousness or encounters with God or a Cosmic Intelligence or even as delusions or, as Bertrand Russell puts it, not rational and real, but only emotional, subjective experiences.

So far as I know, no thinker in modern times has attempted to present 'mystical experience' as an objective reality, as an advanced state of cognition or a wider dimension of consciousness designed for man, not as a harvest of his own manipulations in the form of religious discipline, meditation, yoga, occult practices or any other voluntary effort, but from a still active biological evolution of the brain, which is accelerated or retarded by the mode of life, the way of thinking and the environment of the individual himself. Mystical consciousness is thus a potential, with a biological base, already present in the cerebral structure of man which, in some cases, allows his voluntary efforts to succeed.

I am irresistibly led to this extraordinary conclusion, not only because of my visionary experiences or the series of uncommon events that have occurred in my life, but also because my body, mind and state of perception, as also my thinking, dreams and my creative output all bear witness to the statement I am making, and the conclusions I have drawn after an objective, meticulous study of the phenomenon. This is not all. So far as I know, there is no other one, single rational explanation that can cover the entire range of phenomena connected with the appearance of prophets and enlightened sages in the field of religion and extraordinary geniuses in the province of science, philosophy and arts. There is also no other explanation that can account for the sudden spurts in culture and high jumps in knowledge that occurred in history, at various places, of which the Renaissance in Europe represents the last episode of this kind.

At our present stage of evolution, the human race, including the most intelligent and the most erudite, looks at the universe and her own Self with one eye closed. The other has begun to open, but it may take ages for the lids to part sufficiently to allow every member to have a fuller view of creation, which is lacking at present. I am not making this statement out of the least sense of superiority or pride, but only to clear the confusion that exists, at present, in our thinking, that our knowledge and observation are final and that the world is actually what we perceive it to be or as the latest theories of physicists present it to us.

If the narratives of mystics and enlightened sages, who include among them some of the loftiest figures in history, are to be trusted, and the accounts of the meticulously observed psychic phenomena are to be believed, the world we live in, the objects we perceive, the events we record and the laws which, we believe, rule the universe, are not, in reality, what they seem to be. The inference is clear that we dwell in an enchanted castle, we call the world, which appears real and concrete to us from the basements to the roofs, from the floors to the ceilings, with endless corridors, rooms, halls, attics, doors and windows, true and solid in every fibre and grain. The most minute study of the mammoth structure unfolds level after level and layer after layer, without ever permitting a glimpse of the foundation on which it stands.

We enter this castle at birth and leave it at death under the influence of a spell cast by our brain. When the spell is broken in the mystical trance, the whole colossal creation of magic melts away, revealing a glory behind that no one has been able to portray so far. "The Cibadasa (individual Self) is a product of Maya" says Pancadasi. "Sruti (revelation) and experience both demonstrate that this world is a magical show and Cibadasa is included in it."*

Like the gorgeous palace, built for Aladdin of the Arabian Nights, by the Jinni, a slave to the lamp, the Cosmos is a wondrous piece of magic, conjured up by the wizard we always carry upon our shoulders, namely our brain. Every human being is a prisoner of this most marvellous instrument of magic, fashioned by a stupendous Intelligence, entirely beyond our reach which, by a slight alteration, can present a new vision of the Universe to man. Only a gossamer veil separates the World of Magic from the World of Reality, but we are powerless to remove it without the cooperation of the wizard who holds us in thrall through all the period of our early pilgrimage. Our birth, life and death consist of a procession of events and succession of scenes, wrought by our senses and the mind, out of a stuff of which we have no cognizance at all. Why do we not perceive the world of matter, as it exists—a boundless emptiness, sparsely dotted with minute solar-system-like fields of energy, no one can figure out aright, which our marvellous brain transforms into the infinitely varied wonder-creation we see around.

Why should unintelligent nature contrive this tilt towards deception in the perceptual organs of all animal life on earth, we do not know. Why should our sensory organs, as monitored by the brain, refuse to show the material world, as it basically exists, divested of color, form, shape and size, lent to it by the mind, is a riddle which no one has answered so far. The argument that such a state of perception could not be favourable to the emergence or survival of terrestrial life would be more supportive of the view that there is purpose behind this illusion rather than that chance

* *Pancadasi,* Translation by Swami Swahananda, vii-217

and a blind aimless process of natural selection have been at work in the creation of life.

But, strange to say, we are very little mindful of this 'wizard' dwelling in our head. We do not know why, but of all the organs in the body, our brain receives the least share of our attention. We are reminded of our digestive organs when we eat, of our organs of elimination, when we attend to the call of nature, of our liver and spleen, when we are listless or in a bad mood, of heart and lungs, when we run or climb a height, of our tongue when we taste a delicacy or a bitter medicine, of genitals, when in the ecstacy of love, but, except when racked by a headache, we seldom allow our attention to dwell on the organ to which, more than any other, we owe our very existence, our every thought and every breath.

Countless human beings, every day, when gazing at themselves in a mirror, minutely scan every line and feature to see how they look, when bathing or exercising, carefully survey their limbs, waist and chest to assess the condition of their bodies, when setting out for a function or a banquet glance at themselves up and down to make sure that they look well-groomed and impressive. But either by habit or neglect or an excess of ego, we seldom reflect on the fact that we ourselves and all we know, think, imagine, create, engineer, build, plan or dream of comes from this maryellous piece of bone and flesh about which we think so little and to which we owe so much.

We have become so accustomed to this habit of over-looking the brain that few of us, when working on a book, or a painting or a piece of music or a mechanical device or a problem in science allow their mind to marvel at the amazing device from which all our ideas, inspirations and solutions come. How many of us, I ask, ever reflect on the position that they are mere images cast by a living movie-projector, devised by nature, complete with the panorama they see around, beginning, when the instrument starts to function, at birth, and ending, when it is worn out, beyond repair, at death? How many of those, I repeat, who are proud of their scholarship or talent or of their positions of honor and importance ever remind themselves that they are but thinking shadows projected by a transformed lump of clay—a fragile toy of nature of varied sizes, shapes and degrees of sensitivity, of which billions are made and unmade by her every day?

Perhaps it is the plan of nature that we should not occupy ourselves so much with the brain for the reasons that, if we did so, its incredible complexity and intricacy, which we can never completely grasp, and its mystery, which we can never unravel with our intellect, might cost us such intense thinking and perplexity as could interfere with our efficiency in other spheres of life. An exhaustive study of the brain, carried to the end, could also shatter the delusion, essential for our existence as individuals, that we are somebodies and not merely an agglomerate of the activity of billions of neurons, working tirelessly day and night, at the impulse of a mysterious Force we never perceive, to keep us alive with all our instincts, thoughts, propensities and properties of life.

As even our school books show, every human being carries in his head the controller of the most elaborate communication system, the largest single network of irrigation channels, the most complex of transport arrangements and the most complete chemical laboratory on the earth. Even at this stage of progress and technological advancement, the combined activity of all the more than four billion human beings on this planet, scholars, thinkers, administrators, chemists, engineers, dieticians, farmers, labourers and the rest, is not so well organized as the incalculably varied and exceedingly precise cycle of activity that occurs every moment in the brain. How is it done? Automatically? Unconscious reflexes? Chemical reactions? or what?

O, ingenious man! Formerly, when untutored, it was Spirit, Soul or God. But now, when sophisticated, it is a lifeless agent of some sort. But wherefrom has your own marvellous intelligence which thinks of these answers, come? Has anyone really answered this question so far? Is it forbidden to believe that the universe is run by an Intelligence, a million times more marvellous than ours and, like it, intangible, invisible and incomprehensible? Is it for-

bidden to hold that there are super-conscious forces in the Cosmos of which the knowledge is denied to us? Do we not play a
colossal hoax upon our intelligence, when, with such a huge void
in our knowledge of the very instrument on which our observation and thinking depends, we stick so stubbornly to our views
about ourselves and the world around, while still in the dark
about the mechanism and the accuracy of the instrument itself? I
say this because it is time now for science to fill the gap and to
know more about the breath-taking secrets of the brain.

What an anomaly that, when talking about the formation of
and changes in countless objects around us, the learned, at once,
pour out torrents of words, describing electrons, protons, atoms,
molecules, elements and compounds with their inter-relation-
ships, complete almost to the last detail. When asked about diseases of the body, paint a graphic picture of microbes, viruses,
infection, contagion, vitamin deficiency, lack of iron, calcium or
other elements, insufficient blood, defect in some organ and the
like. But, when talking about distempers of the mind, faults in
thinking and behavior, immoderate desires and passions, uncontrollable anger and hate or irrational fear and depression bring in
a hundred factors to account for the abnormal condition, without
ever mentioning the organ which is inseparably linked with all
that the victims of these distempers experience, suffer, think
or feel.

We never see a full-fledged living mind without a body and we
never see a headless human trunk moving around. The death of
the brain signals the death of the body, the cessation of thought,
feeling and all vital functions that had kept the individual alive, an
active participant in the play of life, with his own individual
characteristics and traits. If a living person sees the dead, it can
only happen through his senses and the mind, while he is alive,
that is in active possession of a living brain. If his communication
with the departed comes about through a medium, it is again the
latter's active brain which makes the connection possible. A dead
medium can no more communicate with a spirit or materialize
one or cause any other phenomena than a log of wood.

All that we know of angels or fairies, devils or demons, whether from actual perception, heresay or study, is the product of some brain, our own or that of someone else. Whatever we hear of magic, sorcery or the occult or of the astral world or of invisible masters and adepts is also the result of someone's experience or thought, again, through the agency of the cranial matter. What does not emerge out of it we never know. What it does not show, we never perceive. What it cannot think of we never conceive.

There never has existed a living human being with exceptional talents, paranormal gifts or spiritual insights without a brain. And, as we have seen, even a discarnate mind needs the brain of a living person to manifest itself. If it is so, why do we always harp on mind and soul without casting even a side glance at that which is indispensible for their activity, as the eye is for one's sight? When there is the slightest impairment in one's vision, the eyeball at once comes in for examination and discussion and we are advised not to lose a minute in these preliminaries. But, when there is even a glaring abnormality in our habits, thinking or behaviour, how many psychologists or psychiatrists begin with an examination of the encephalon, even from external signs, and how many of them are even capable of doing so?

The erudite, when they wax eloquent on the human mind, describing its nooks and corners, heights and depressions, desires and ambitions, loves and hates, fancies and dreams, tensions and distractions or illnesses and ailments, except in the case of brain diseases, often give a wide berth to this organ, as if it is irrelevant to the discussion and prudently confine themselves only to that which is the easier of the two to dwell on. In the same way, the ecclesiastics, the divines, spiritual preceptors, masters, adepts and yogis, who pose as authorities in man's search for the Divine, cautiously refrain from the least reference to the cranium, as if it does not come into the picture at all. What a strange perversity of the human ego that, while completely in the dark about the source from which its thinking and imagination, if not its very life comes, it should strut and dance on the stage of human achievement, in every field, arrogating every ounce of credit to itself until hurled into oblivion by a failure of the same mechanism on which it had not even deigned to cast a look.

The assumption that every human being possesses a soul does not materially affect the position. In fact, the very idea of soul is a creation of our mind. If it is argued that soul is the mind or that mind is an instrument of the soul, in either case the argument does not, in any way, detract from the importance of the brain. Whether soul is the master of the body or the mind, whether they are one or separate, the brain is the vehicle of their manifestation, the seat of their activity and the ground for their existence in the embodied form. When there is no brain, the soul or mind cease to be active participants in the dream of life.

We do not know what the soul looks like nor where the mind comes from. All that we know is that we are clothed in a body, with hands to work with and feet to move about, with senses to perceive the outer world and a brain to know, think with and exercise control over them all. Who can deny that we are only what our brain makes us, intelligent or stupid, irascible or wild, cunning or artless, wicked or good, lustful or temperate and the rest, invested by it with varied traits of character or, at least, with a predisposition for them, often from birth! Our composite personality cannot survive even a moment when the brain is dead. We do not know what makes the whole personality of an individual change suddenly for the better or for worse, under certain conditions, as for instance in spontaneous religious conversions, sudden bursts of illumination, in a crisis, under a shock and the like. In such cases, some kind of upheaval must be occurring in the brain because what happens to the personality must be the imprint of a parallel occurrence there. But the secret of how these well-authenticated transformations occur is still unknown.

We are gradually coming to realize that the visible and tangible world around us, with its mountains, oceans, deserts, plains, sun and moon, animals and plants is only a world of sensations caused by the impact of an indefinable energy on the antennae of our senses, protruding from the brain, and all that we see, hear, touch, taste and smell is the result of the contact of these two indeterminable elements, mind and a colorless, tasteless, odorless, soundless and formless sea of energy and nothing more. What then creates the marvellous world of endless colors, sounds, smells, flavors and forms round us?

We have no answer to this question yet. The very idea that the brain can take a leap and change not only the personality, but the entire picture of the Universe, in the case of some individuals, will appear novel to many people. It is hard to believe that the human brain is changing imperceptibly and with that the picture of the Universe as also the personality of man are undergoing a transformation. The reason for this is rooted in the fact that a wall of silence surrounds our organ of thought, except for scattered bits of information here and there. This silence remains unbroken for the reason that the scholar, scientist or philosopher who breaks it, must have the courage to confess that the ideas he has expressed on some subject, some aspect of philosophy or some issue of science are only tentative, subject to modification or confirmation on a fuller knowledge of the brain! I say this because with the next spurt in the knowledge of the cerebral cortex, not distant now, a good many tall edifices in philosophy, psychology and even other branches of science will come toppling down to the earth.

I have a strong reason for making this statement, for with the first successful exploratory survey of the brain, a revolution will occur in certain vital areas of human knowledge that would put into shade the giant revolutions caused by the modern cosmogenal concepts of science. The first harvest of this revolution will be the discovery for us of the intangible Cosmic Element behind the phenomena of life. It would prove to be a hundred times more difficult task to give a name and form to this ineffable Source than what science is facing at the moment in giving a precise definition and form to matter at the finer levels at which it is being studied now. In fact, the indeterminacy and nebulosity which science is encountering betokens the last limit to which the human sensory equipment and intellect can guide it. Beyond that another faculty must come into operation to show the position of the same world, when viewed from another level of consciousness. It is only the study of the cosmic panorama, done through this new channel of perception, that can correct the errors made in the survey done before.

Secondly, the very idea of continued evolution carries with it the conditon that, in the more evolved state, the transfigured specimens will be, in some way, mentally more advanced than the rest with other faculties and intellectual gifts not possessed by the common ranks, however intelligent they might be. Were it possible for the human wit to solve all the riddles by which she is surrounded, there would arise no need for further evolution nor would there remain any incentive for individuals to apply themselves to the difficult task of transcending the present state. This is what a more advanced knowledge of the brain would make clear. The impassable frontiers now reached by science, the disaffection with the prevailing political orders of the earth and the shortcomings of current faiths, coupled with the widening perspectives of leading scientists, the fast awakening political consciousness in the masses everywhere and the growing urge for self-awareness in the rising generations, will soon make the existence of a wiser and more perspicacious rank of leading men and women, perceptive of the super-sensory world, imperative for the race to instruct and guide her in the knowledge of both the Kingdoms—the one we live in and the other to come.

There is no doubt that many among the readers of this book would exhibit surprise at the assurance I display in flinging a challenge to the learned assemblies of the earth. If I did not do so, and fail to vindicate my stand, all my talk about the extraordinary nature of the experience I have undergone, the insight I have gained, the knowledge I have gathered, the paranormal gifts I have won, and the advanced state of perception I have acquired would be mere idle prattle, a condemnable string of untruths, woven into a concocted tale, like scores of other fictitious stories about the supernatural which hit the high-water mark during recent years.

I was poorly educated and, as compared to the giants of learning of our time, am deplorably short of knowledge of arts and science. Penury dogged my footsteps from the day I was born to the time I was grey with age. Apart from this, my abrupt entry into the paranormal took the form of a perilous adventure that carried me, a complete stranger, along a highly steep, tortuous and slippery mountain path to the ridge of a summit, where I precariously dwell, at present, in a glittering fairyland, with yawning chasms on either side. How I live, with this unheard of but easily discernible change in my nervous system, I am myself at a loss to understand.

But, even with all these gruelling ordeals, I have emerged triumphant, with an ample share of happiness, above all the pleasures of earth, and an insight into a mystery which, when solved, can throw a flood of light on some of the still unsolved riddles of the mind and pave the way to a better understanding of the human destiny and a more harmonious and joyful future for the human society which she, without the Midas touch of this knowledge, cannot hope to attain. I feel confident, because the secret has been tried, and I am myself a minor product of this trial. I could never have shared this knowledge with others had not my brain, almost by a miracle, time and again, stood well the hammering which it received, while I helplessly watched the pounding day and night. To those who feel outraged by my presumption, I can only say in all humility, that it is not I, but the unerring hand of providence that would bring about this consummation, to divert the course of human effort, which has become aberrant, in the right direction consistent with the future destiny of the race.

An oculist, professing ability to cure disease of the eyes, enhance their performance, or improve sight, must have a good knowledge of their anatomy and physiology, of the nerves which line them, the optical center in the brain, the bodily conditions which adversely affect their functioning and the rest. Without this knowledge, he would be called a quack. He can then no more call himself an oculist than a plumber, without even the rudiments of medical knowledge, can call himself a physician. In treating the eyes, the oculist must possess a clear knowledge of errors, faults and diseases peculiar to the eye. He must know when people need glasses to correct their vision in middle age, that many cannot distinguish all the colors and some only a few, that there are people who cannot distinguish objects at night and the like.

In the same way, those who profess to be proficient in the science of mind must have at least a passing knowledge of the inter-relationship between brain and thought. If this is lacking, the views expressed about mind, as also about its eccentric or abnormal behavior, by any acknowledged authority, cannot be accepted as scientific, for the simple reason that the faults noticed might be due to impurities in the organic filter, that is the brain, which cloud the transparency of the intangible stuff whereof thought is made, and not to flaws in the stuff itself. Such views would be like the mythical explanations provided for the phases of the moon in ancient times, before the real reasons for its waxing and waning were known.

We know very well how deceptive our eyes can be. They clearly see the sun moving in the sky, rising in the East and setting in the West. They see the stars change their position in the sky at night, and the moon sailing across it, waxing and waning, from a barely visible thin crescent to a full orb and back again to the crescent form. They see objects looking smaller at a distance, diminishing in size as they move further and further away, until they become too small to be distinguished. They see the dome of the sky meeting the earth, all around, at a certain distance, the junction point extending further and further as they climb a height and growing narrower and narrower as they descend.

The disk of the colossal sun, thousands of times the size of the earth, appears to them no larger than the disk of a coin held close to the eye. We know that for many thousands of years human beings implicitly believed in the evidence of their eyes, and framed their picture of the earth and the universe round them accordingly. We also know what a radical change has been wrought in the thinking and ideas of mankind with the advent of the telescope and the microscope. How many errors have been corrected, how many delusions cleared and how many new worlds, both macroscopic and microscopic, have been opened before our eyes, about which our own great-grandparents and thousands of generations before them had no idea at all.

We are slowly overcoming the deceptive appearances presented by our eyes, extending their power and range with instruments, and thereby gaining more and more knowledge of the wonders of the sky, the marvels of microscopic life and ultra-microscopic levels of matter, that were never even thought of before. Even the wisest of antiquity had no knowledge of what the children of our age know and talk about freely. No sensible person can deny that even the most venerated sages and prophets of the past could not conceive of the wonders that are a common sight for us today.

Plato, Aristotle or Vyasa had no idea that glasses and hearing aids could keep white-haired men and women as mentally alert and responsive as they are now. In fact, the average age-span during those days was much shorter than it is now. After them, Patanjali, Galen or Aviceena had no inkling that eyes, heart or kidneys could be transplanted or that human life could be possible on one kidney alone. Similarly, Tulsi Dass, Saidi, Dante and Milton could never imagine that one in Persia could listen instantaneously to a conversation carried on in Paris, as distinctly as if it was being held in the next room. It is not hard to conceive that our not too distant progeny might be taught in schools what is beyond the reach of even the most brilliant minds of our day. There are wide gaps in our knowledge on every side which the future is bound to fill. This is particularly true of the brain. The learned, who believe in the finality of their views, would do well to remember that their future generation of descendants, in their very teens, would know more about the world than what they do now, at the end of a long life devoted to study day and night.

How can we know that the brain does not deceive us in the same way as the eyes do? In fact, strictly speaking, the former must be a party to the deception practiced by the sensory organs, whether eyes or ears. How can we know that in other matters, too, our brain does not act in the same way as our senses, keeping some planes of creation hidden from us, and presenting disguised and distorted pictures of others to create the illusion of the world we live in. Our ears reveal to us only a fragment of the world of sound, our eyes only a thin section of the world of sight, our nose and tongue only a fraction of the world of smell and taste. Since our brain must be a party to this manipulation, in the case of every sensual organ which we own, it is obvious, there must be some reason why living creatures are allowed only a limited range of perception which makes the world appear as we see it and not as our instruments reveal it to be.

Based on his own experiences, Bucke postulated evolution as the factor responsible for mystical experience. As far as I know, no one of the few psychologists who made mysticism a subject of their study, after him, caught the hint to proceed further in the investigation. One of the reasons for this could be the singularity of the idea and the second, complete lack of corroboration from biologists. Since specialization of knowledge has made it penal for the experts in one discipline to encroach upon the territory of the other, the idea did not catch fire. Some idea of what I mean can be gathered from Huxley's Introduction to Teilhard de Chardin's *The Phenomenon of Man*.

There is a high degree of acuteness of certain senses in some creatures, as for instance dogs, migratory birds, bees, moths, whales, etc. which is out of reach of the others. Again, an enigma of the brain! Most of the animals do not possess color vision. As Bucke has shown, the sense of color is a comparatively recent acquisition of the human race. But even at this stage all human beings are not equally sensitive to color. "We have the authority of Max Mueller," writes Bucke, "for the statement that Xenophanes knew of three colors of the rainbow only—purple, red and yellow; that even Aristotle spoke of the tri-colored rainbow; and that Democritus knew of no more than four colors—black, white, red and yellow. Geiger points out that it can be proved by examination of language that, as late in the life of the race as the time of the primitive Aryans, perhaps, not more than fifteen or twenty thousand years ago, man was only conscious of, only perceived, one color. That is to say, he did not distinguish any difference in tint between the blue sky, the green trees and grass, the brown or grey earth, and the golden and purple clouds of sunrise and sunset. So Pictet finds no names of colors in primitive Indo-European speech. And Max Mueller finds no Sanskrit root whose meaning has any reference to color. Still later, at the time when the bulk of the Rig Veda was composed, red, yellow and black were recognized as three separate shades, but these three included all color that man at that age was capable of appreciating."*

"In no part of the world" continues Bucke, "is the blue of the sky more intense than in Greece and Asia Minor, where the Homeric poems were composed. Is it possible to conceive that a poet (or the poets) who saw this, as we see it now, could write the forty-eight long books of the Iliad and Odyssey and never once either mention or refer to it? But were it possible that all the poets of the Rig Veda, Zend Avesta, Iliad, Odyssey and Bible could have omitted the mention of the blue color of the sky by mere accident, etymology would step in and assure us that four thousand years ago or, perhaps, three, blue was unknown, for at that time the subsequent names for blue were all merged in the names for black."

The sense of fragrance seems to have developed even later. "Another recently acquired faculty" says Bucke, "is the sense of fragrance. It is not mentioned in the Vedic hymns and only once in the Zend Avesta." *Musical sense, in the opinion of Bucke, has existed for less than (perhaps considerably less than) five thousand years and it does not exist in more than half the members of the race. He adduces these recent additions to human sensibility as evidence of human evolution and moral progress. How can we fit in all this in an organically static brain? The merest shred of evidence to show that the human cerebral cortex is still in the process of evolution opens up a field of enquiry so important that it should have received a hundredfold more urgent attention than

---

* R. M. Bucke, *Cosmic Consciousness*
* Ibid

the present-day spectacular, but highly extravagant enterprise for the exploration of distant planets aimed, at the best, to satisfy a curiosity and not, as in the case of the former, to gather new knowledge essential for the welfare and survival of the race.

From this it is easy to infer how the world must have appeared to our ancestors thirty or only twenty thousand years ago—a world devoid of the rich variety of color, captivating melody of sounds and the lovely blend of perfumes which delight our senses today. The inner world, too, of the primitives of that time must have been almost empty of the sense of beauty, symmetry, loveliness and grace which ravish our mind and the ideas of goodness, purity, chivalry, compassion, nobility and unselfish love which inspire us today. If at all present, they must have existed only in extremely feeble, inchoate forms. If the human mind continues to grow richer and richer in sensory perception and more and more imbued with lofty ideas and noble sentiments, as has imperceptibly happened in the past, what kind of man should we expect, at the present extremely slow pace of progress, say after ten thousand years?

On the basis of the transformation that has already occurred in our mental equipment, it should not be very difficult to draw a fairly close imaginary picture of the man to come. If we do so and compare it with that of one of the great mystics of the past, after a study of the latter's life, strivings, ideals, sacrifices, rich visionary experiences and the transporting world unfolded within, we cannot but be struck by the points of resemblance between the two. Divest the picture of religiosity, doctrinal coloring, extreme asceticism and penance, dogma and superstition and you have before you a hazy portrait of the future man or woman, rich in the wealth of the soul, with high ideals and noblest qualities of the head and the heart. We will find so much to distinguish them from the average worldly-minded individual of our day that the time-lag of centuries between the two will at once become apparent.

Our primitive ancestor did not perceive the same world which our senses present to us today, embellished with color, fragrance, symphony and a hundred other things which did not at all form a part of his spirit-infested, superstition-filled, dull, sordid, color-less world. It is not surprising that he fashioned his deities or their hideous, repulsive visages in images and idols in the likeness of his own savage mind and the forbidding prospect he saw around by the poverty of his own instrument of perception. In the same way our distant progeny, turning back the pages of history, will mark our faults, foibles and lacks, as we mark them in our remote ancestors, conscious of and thankful for the wide gulf which now separates us from them.

I do not say this with any intent to belittle the achievements of our time, but only to remind those who think too highly of their learning, looks, position, color, caste, pedigree or ethnic type that our uncouth predecessors, who now appear so primitive to our eyes, must have felt the same way, swelling with pride and beaming with satisfaction at their own limited knowledge, impor-tance, prowess or the genealogy of their tribe in the world envi-ronment in which they lived. It is not the breath-taking innovations in the mechanical wonders of today, which the science-fiction writers paint so gaudily, that would matter so much in the times ahead, as the change in the thinking and perception of man him-self. The world is in darkness about a momentous secret, as vital for its existence as the air we breathe; but the learned, over-confident of their scholarship and, too often, suspicious of reli-gion, fail to enlighten us, prevented from penetrating to the Truth by the veil of pride interposed by Destiny.

3

Consciousness and Super Consciousness

In the preceding chapters I have tried to show, firstly, that the number of the mystics who had the genuine experience, throughout the course of history, has been extremely small, and that all those who claim knowledge of the spirit are not really enlightened. Secondly, that the present world is woefully deficient in the knowledge of the brain and that the learned, in dealing with mind or the origin and nature of the universe, usually leave the encephalon out of count, as if human intelligence exists incorporeally and independently, and does not depend for its manifestation, quality and performance on the activity of an organic instrument, beyond our scrutiny at present. The result is that much of our knowledge, at the moment, is unilateral and speculative, nescient of the nature of the 'Knower' itself. An intelligent species with a brain that shows an altered perception of time, an easy possibility, would frame an entirely different picture of the universe.

The aim of this writing is to draw attention to this serious lacunae which keeps us in ignorance about our own selves. The position that I am taking up is that the human mind, as we know it at present, is not a constant, unalterable entity. It can change and with it the whole picture of the universe, which we perceive with our senses. This is a bold statement to make, and is not likely to be accepted for the simple reason that it undermines the very foundation on which science is built, namely, the reality of the objective world and the validity of the empirical observation conducted by the mind.

The issue boils down to this: if it is admitted that the human mind is variable and that this variation can affect the very image of the universe, and all the phenomena observed, it would clearly imply that the cosmos is not, in reality, as we perceive, assess and measure it with our intelligence, but only a creation of our mind liable to change in other dimensions of the perceptive faculty. From this it would follow that the temporal knowledge gathered by us is relative also and that what is accumulated in one dimension of consciousness can prove incomplete, deceptive or erroneous in the other.

"Our conception of the structure of the Universe," says William de Sitter, "bears all the marks of a transitory structure. Our theories are decidedly in a state of continuous, and just now very rapid evolution. It is not possible to predict how long our present views and interpretations will remain unaltered and how soon they will have to be replaced by perhaps very different ones, based on new observational data and new critical insight in their connection with other data."* Where from is this new critical insight to come except from a more evolved mind and brain?

An affirmation of the same position comes from no less than an authority than Max Planck. He says: "How do we discover the individual laws of Physics, and what is their nature? It should be remarked, to begin with, that we have no right to assume that any physical laws exist, or if they have existed up to now, that they will continue to exist in a similar manner in the future. It is perfectly conceivable that one fine day Nature should cause an unexpected event to occur which would baffle us all; and if this were to hap-

---

* William de Sitter, *Relativity and Modern Theories of the Universe*

pen we would be powerless to make any objection, even if the result would be that, in spite of our endeavors, we should fail to introduce order into the resulting confusion. In such an event, the only course open to science would be to declare itself bankrupt. For this reason, science is compelled to begin by the general assumption that a general rule of law dominates throughout Nature."*

Once the position is accepted, the conclusion becomes unavoidable that all the contexts of our day-to-day experience of the world—the events which befall and the sights we see, the good and evil, noble and base, beautiful and ugly we meet, or the ideas of God, Soul and the Hereafter we entertain, all emerge from the unfathomable depths of our consciousness. This means that all we come across during the pilgrimage of life is not an objective reality, but a stupendous, realistic drama, presented by our own mind, and another enigmatic stuff, we call material energy. The latter is becoming more and more of a paradox and the more we try to reach its bottom the more paradoxical and unpredictable it becomes. For all we know, it might be a twin brother of our mind, both off-shoots of the same tree or a projected image of mind itself. The corollary that follows this view of creation, forced on us by the latest concepts in physics, is that since our brain is the junction-point, where this incredible exchange between the mind and his brother takes place, it is to the brain that we must look for a solution of the mystery.

The matter does not end there. What should now become obvious, beyond doubt, is the fact that when contemplating a grand spectacle of nature, during the day, or the shimmering firmament at night, the sense of admiration, awe or wonder felt does not come from the magnificence, loveliness or the vast extent of these external objects, inherent or dwelling in them, but from the grandeur, beauty and the immensity residing in our own consciousness. In other words, it is we who lend grandiosity, charm

---

* Max Planck, *Universe in the Light of Modern Physics*

and vastness to an object, also horror, cheerfulness, humor or sadness to what appears to us as a dreadful, merry, ludicrous or tragic scene. What the world will look like to a mind, dead to emotions and bereft of the sense of beauty and color, I leave it to the reader to imagine.

This still does not complete the picture. The other conclusion that follows is that all the over four billion human creatures on the earth, the multi-millionaire and the pauper, the king and the beggar, the strongman and the cripple, the philanthropist and the thief, the beauty-queen and the leper, as long as they live, share the same incredible wonder in their interior, as they share the sun, the moon, the stars, the air and water, the precious bounties of nature that make life possible on earth.

It is a staggering position. But there is nothing incongruous in what I say. The scriptures of all the current faiths point to the same conclusion. Since the Soul is held to be immortal, incorporeal and divine, it must always stay immaculate, above the corporeality and the blemishes of the mortal frame. It would be blasphemous to say that there can be a sightless, lecherous, leprous or penniless Soul. It is because of an impure frame of mind which attaches more importance to the externals of religion than to its beatific interior that we are denied access to the Glory that dwells in all of us, irrespective of our station in life.

The main task of religion is to bring awareness of the divinity within to every human being. In this unique treasure of heaven no one is richer, stronger, superior or better than the other. This divine Splendor all share alike, irrespective of their position, wealth, learning, intelligence, strength or looks. Like the brilliant orb of the day, it shines alike on the rich and the poor, the wise and the fool. The glaring differences and discrepencies, elegance and squalor, virture and vice or excess and want we see around, belong to the stage and the dress of clay and not to the divine actor, ever undefiled, like a dancing beam of light. The aim of human life is to explore this 'wonder' in every one of us whose pleasure-ground is the universe.

This is the Message which for the last over three thousand

years the exalted class of true mystics has brought to the world. This is the Message which juvenile science, at first, cared not to heed like an impetuous youngster refusing to listen to his more seasoned elders, ultimately in his declining age to regret the rebellious thoughts of his early years. There are myriads who, in their closing days, review with sorrow their reckless youth. Were there no surprises and no innovations in the province of thought in store for the human wit in the ages to come, she would die of boredom in a few centuries. It is change that keeps her alive. The pendulum is now swinging in the other direction to usher in a new era of thought in which the spirit and not matter, the mystic and not the skeptic will dominate.

An indication of this change is provided by the thoughts expressed by many eminent scientists of recent times. This is a sample of one of them: "Yet I repeat once more," declares William James, "the existence of mystical states absolutely overthrows the pretention of non-mystical states to be the sole and ultimate dictators of what we may believe. As a rule, mystical states merely add a super-sensuous meaning to the ordinary outward data of consciousness. They are excitements, like the emotions of love or ambition, gifts to our spirit by means of which facts, already objectively before us, fall into a new expressiveness and make a new connection with our active life. They do not contradict these facts as such, or deny anything that our senses have immediately seized. It is the rationalistic critic rather who plays the part of denier in the controversy, and his denials have no strength, for there can never be a state of facts to which new meaning may not truthfully be added, provided the mind ascends to a more envelop-ing point of view. It must always remain an open question whether mystical states may not possibly be such superior points of view, windows through which the mind looks out upon a more exten-sive and inclusive world."*

The present-day concepts of physics no longer contradict the

---

* William James, *The Varieties of Religious Experience*

experience of the mystic but, on the other hand, find it more consistent with the new insights into the nature of the physical world. This view has been expressed by many among the leading physicists of our time. "A rainbow described in the symbolism of physics," writes Eddington, "is a band of aethereal vibrations arranged in systemic order to wave-lengths from about .00004 centimeters to .000072 centimeters. From one point of view, we are paltering with the truth whenever we admire the gorgeous bow of color, and should strive to reduce our minds to such a state that we receive the same impression from the rainbow as from a table of wave-lengths. But although that is how the rainbow impresses itself on an impersonal spectroscope, we are not giving the whole truth and significance of experience—the starting-point of the problem—if we suppress the factors wherein we ourselves differ from the spectroscope. We cannot say that the rainbow, as part of the world, was meant to convey the vivid effects of color; but we can perhaps say that the human mind, as part of the world, was meant to perceive it that way."*

Another eminent physicist, James Jeans writes, "In more recent times, Bertrand Russell has expressed what is essentially the same argument in the words: 'So long as we adhere to the conventional notions of mind and matter, we are condemned to a view of perception which is miraculous. We suppose that a physical process starts from a visible object, travels to the eye, there changes into another physical process, causes yet another physical process in the optic nerve, and finally produces some effect in the brain, simultaneously with which we see the object from which the process started, the seeing being something "mental," totally different in character from the physical processes which precede and accompany it.' This view is so queer that metaphysicians have invented all sorts of theories designed to substitute something less incredible...

"Everything that we can directly observe of the physical world

---

* A. S. Eddington, *Science and Mysticism*

happens inside our heads, and consists of mental events which form part of the physical world. The development of this point of view will lead us to the conclusion that the distinction between mind and matter is illusory. The stuff of the world may be called physical or mental or both or neither as we please; in fact the words serve no purpose."*

"Even if the two entities which we have hitherto described," continues Jeans, "as mind and matter are of the same general nature, there remains the question as to which is the more fundamental of the two. Is mind only a by-product of matter, as the materialists claimed? Or is it, as Berkeley claimed, the creator and controller of matter?

"Before the latter alternative can be seriously considered, some answer must be found to the problem of how objects can continue to exist when they are not being perceived in any human mind. There must, as Berkeley says, be 'some other mind in which they exist.' Some will wish to describe this, with Berkeley, as the mind of God; others with Hegel as a universal or Absolute mind in which all our individual minds are comprised. The new quantum mechanics may perhaps give a hint, although nothing more than a hint, as to how this can be."*

"It seems, at least, conceivable," Jeans adds, "That what is true of perceived objects may also be true of perceiving minds; just as there are wave-pictures for light and electricity, so there may be a corresponding picture for consciousness. When we view ourselves in space and time, our consciousness is obviously the separate individuals of a particle-picture, but when we pass beyond space and time, they may perhaps form ingredients of a single continuous stream of life. As it is with light and electricity, so it may be with life; the phenomena may be individuals carrying on separate existences in space and time, while in the deeper reality beyond space and time we may all be members of one body. In brief, modern physics is not altogether antagonistic to an objec-

---

* James Jeans, *Some Problems of Philosophy*
* Ibid

tive idealism like that of Hegel."*

I know it will be hard for me to make myself understood, as I tread on unmapped territory in the effort to bring into focus in the province of religion and science both, a vital element that has been ignored so far, namely, the center of life in the body, that is the brain. Since the organ is indispensible for all our activity and even existence in the human form, it is inconceivable that our consciousness can take a leap beyond its normal periphery without affecting its substance in any way. There is no historical precedent of a higher animal, say a horse, ever attaining the mental stature of a human being, and co-mingling with other humans on a basis of equality. How can it then be possible for a human being to consort with gods without some kind of change in the brain? Those who long for self-awareness, clairvoyant gifts, miraculous powers, communication with the spirit world, encounters with masters, or adventures in the occult realm would do well to give second thoughts to their cherished dream. The world did not produce another Christ or Buddha, Vyasa or Socrates, Plato or Mohammed, Rumi or Shankaracharya, Francis of Assisi or any other great mystic or master of the occult, because the mystery of the part played by the brain in these accomplishments remains unsolved so far. The aim of this writing is to make this hidden knowledge accessible to humanity.

I am confident of my stand, as a psychological cathartic is necessary to crown the revolution caused by science, and its off-spring, technology, in human life and thought. Without this psychological climax, mankind will continue to move in the accustomed groove and utilize the resources of the earth and also of her fertile intellect only to enhance and satisfy her physical needs as she is virtually doing now. Her most pressing need at the moment is to become aware of the spiritual goal planned for her by nature and the methods to attain it. Once this knowledge is gained and the unmatched splendor of the crown destined for her realized,

* Ibid

no efforts of pharisees or saddusees, who thrive on the credulity and naivity of human beings, can make the race deviate from the course.

A tidal wave of skepticism, doubt and disbelief, symbolized by the materialist ideology, is sweeping over the earth, not because Satan and the Anti-Christ have become dominant nor because it is Kali-Yuga of the Indian mythology, but because the time for a further elaboration and enrichment of the religious creeds and spiritual ideals of mankind has come. Like a cocoon, man weaves a tough sheet of dogma around himself to lie inert and passive until nature tears it open with a revolution to allow him freedom. But he soon starts to weave it afresh in the newly introduced pattern of life or thought to entomb himself once again. This is true not only of religion but also of political orders, social customs, educational systems, even scientific institutions and other long-standing ideas and beliefs. It is easier, sometimes, to bore a tunnel through a mountain than to break open the shell which the conservative element in human nature builds round itself.

To believe that the universe consists of only those elements and forces that are perceptible to our senses or detected by our instruments is to belie the latest assessments of science. The very size and the extent of the Universe, the new formations discovered in the sky and the problems created by them, the marvels of the ultra-microscopic world and the possibility of even superior types of life in other parts of the Cosmos provide more than sufficient material to make it clear that the creation round us is too complex, too vast and too full of unsolved riddles to make us complacent about the fact that what our senses perceive or minds apprehend is all that exists in it. Such an attitude of mind at this stage of our knowledge can only emanate from one not in touch with the progress of today.

The first impact of genuine mystical experience on the mind of the experiencer is something like this - that the world he was perceiving and his own individuality, as he was conscious of it so far, were not true realities but only the figures of, say, a relative speaking, dream state from which he has just awakened to the full blaze of another sun shining on a splendrous world, entirely unlike the one which his senses were revealing to him before. It should be remembered that for this state of cognition, it is not necessary that the percipient should be insensible to the sensory world. Not at all. What makes mystical ecstasy an increasing wonder is the incredible fact that both the sensory and supersensory worlds can be perceived simultaneously. But how? Like the radiant sky showing a mirage on it, both visible side by side.

The real status of the 'mystic' has not been correctly adjudged so far. He is not a dreamy idealist prone to visions, conjured up by his subconscious or to epileptic seizures or to hysterical swoons or to ecstatic trances, brought about by a suppressed libido, or his own obsessive occupation with the supernatural or by a pathological condition of the brain. In those cases, where these symptoms have been exhibited by true mystics, the abnormalities were the concomitant features of the extraordinary mental state, as in the case of genius, and not the causative factors responsible for it. These are mere conjectures of the learned made in absence of an accurate knowledge of the phenomenon. Nor is he a special protege of the Almighty, sent to the earth to preach His glory among mortals and to exhort them to surrender their all for His sake and, himself intoxicated with His love, to infuse this intoxication in others also. The human intellect has since outgrown the anthropomorphic picture of the Creator and it is time she outgrows the current picture of the mystic too.

Every mystic born has been a specimen of the man to come. His self-imposed penances and his religious beliefs were the creation of his culture, faith and the environment around him. But his vivid descriptions of the new visions gained, the new worlds unfolded and his basic teachings about the way to be followed to reach the same state of perception were the outcome of knowledge gained in the new dimension of consciousness to which he had attained. The descriptions are diversely colored and at times contradictory and conflicting because they are, as it were, the first reports of a few space travellers, separated by long stretches of time and distance, viewing the gigantic planet, Jupiter, at a distance of hundreds of thousands of miles from different angles through glasses of varied magnifying power.

Nature repeatedly produced the prototype of the future man to awaken humanity to her destiny. But the multitudes, including the scholars and the divines, misinterpreting the hint, erected for themselves the four walls of ritualistic religions to confine themselves within, with a fanatical zeal which led to some of the greatest horrors in history, still repeated at times in some parts of the earth. That the followers of every faith arrogate to their own creed the highest station among all the religions, to their founder or founders the highest stature among all the prophets and to themselves the most favored position with the Almighty, makes it obvious that the human ego has been as strongly at work in this holy territory, where humility is the law, as in the other spheres of life. This shows that self-worshipping man does not even spare his Maker in the fulfillment of his selfish ends and makes of Him, too, a tool to bolster his own vanity.

I have purposely introduced the prosaic figure of the human brain in this discourse to serve as an anchor to the otherwise highly mobile vessel of thought, prone to be carried away here and there by the wind of prejudice, dogma, idiosyncrasy, stubbornness and the rest, especially when sailing on the waters of religion, philosophy or metaphysics. It is only experiments on the brain that can call a dead halt to these arbitrary flights of human thought when dealing with the phenomena of mind. In order to explain why this need has arisen, I can do no better than refer the reader to the views expressed by some of the writers on mysticism in recent times. For instance, Evelyn Underhill, in answering for her self-formulated question, "What then is the nature of this special sense—this transcendental consciousness—and how does contemplation liberate it," proceeds to explain:

"Any attempt to answer this question brings upon the scene another aspect of man's psychic life: an aspect of paramount importance to the student of the mystic type. We have reviewed the chief ways in which our surface consciousness reacts upon experience: a surface consciousness which has been trained through long ages to deal with the universe of sense. We know, however, that the personality of man is a far deeper and more mysterious thing than the sum of his conscious feeling, thought and will: that this superficial self—this Ego of which each of us is aware—hardly counts in comparison with the depths of being which it hides. 'There is a root or depth in Thee,' says Law, 'from whence all these faculties come forth as lines from a center, or branches from the body of a tree. This depth is called the center, the fund, or bottom of the soul. This depth is the unity, the Eternity, I had almost said the infinity of the soul, for it is so infinite that nothing can satisfy it or give it any rest, but the infinity of God.' "*

"Since normal man is utterly unable to set up relations with spiritual reality by means of his feeling, thought and will," continues Underhill, "it is clearly in this depth of being—in these unplumbed levels of personality—that we must search if we would find the organ, the power, by which he is to achieve the mystic quest. The alteration of consciousness which takes place in contemplation can only mean the emergence from this 'fund or bottom of the soul' of some faculty which diurnal life keeps hidden 'in the deeps.'"*

To draw a parallel for her own conclusion, Underhill turns to the widely used concept of the 'unconscious mind,' a handy device of modern psychology to explain whatever is unexplainable or unintelligible in the area of mind. "Modern psychology," she continues, "in its doctrine of the unconscious or subliminal personality, has acknowledged this fact of a range of psychic life, lying below and beyond the conscious field. Indeed, it has so dwelt upon and defined this shadowy region—which is really less a 'region' than a useful name—that it sometimes seems to know more about the unconscious than about the conscious life of man. There it finds, side by side, the sources of his most animal instincts, his least explicable powers, his most spiritual intuitions:

---

* Evelyn Underhill, *Mysticism*
* Ibid

the 'ape and tiger,' and the 'soul.' Genius and prophecy, insomnia and infatuation, clairvoyance, hypnotism, hysteria and 'Christian' science—all are explained by the 'unconscious mind.' In his destructive moods, the psychologist has little apparent difficulty in reducing the chief phenomena of religious and mystical experience to activities of the 'unconscious,' seeking an oblique satisfaction of repressed desires. Where he undertakes the more dangerous duties of apologetic, he explains the same phenomena by saying that 'God speaks to man in the subconscious,' by which he can only mean that our apprehension of the eternal has the character of intuition rather than of thought. Yet the 'unconscious' after all is merely a convenient name for the aggregate of those powers, parts or qualities of the whole self which at any given moment are not conscious or that the Ego is not conscious of."*

I have reproduced these passages at some length for two reasons. Firstly, to show the similarity between my ideas and the view expressed that mystical vision is the herald of a 'new birth,' the symbol of a profound transformation in the personality of an individual which reaches down to the roots of his being, making him perceptive of spiritual realities denied to the average human folk. Secondly, to bring into focus the usual tendency among modern writers on religion, metaphysics or psychology to keep out the brain in their discussion as if it does not come into the picture at all. This habit allows too loose a rein to fancy. We know very well that even a slight alteration in the chemistry of the brain, brought about by a drug, a shock or loss of sleep can cause an explosive change in consciousness or the personality of the subject for the time being. Hence to suppose that such a signal event as the experience of God or the entry into supersensory planes of creation can be possible without involving the cranial matter in any way is but to confess the fault, now common among scholars, of dissociating thought from the brain, both inseparable chums

---

* Ibid

from birth to death.

The answer to Underhill comes very near to the commonly accepted explanations for the extraordinary experience of mystics and saints. The notion is that there are submerged capacities and potentialities in the human soul which can make these enrapturing flights to the holy precincts of divine consciousness possible for those who apply themselves heart and soul to the task. Linked inextricably to the idea that mystical ecstasy represents a union with or, at least, a vision of God, and that the human soul is a particle of the divine essence, an explanation of this kind has every semblance of plausibility and usually puts the doubts of the enquirer to rest.

Every human being is aware of himself as a self-contained independent unit of consciousness. The brain does not protrude into the personality at all. For this reason, we do not think of it any more than of other parts of the body and at times, even less. On account of the fact that a serious injury to the head can easily prove fatal, all that the people exposed to accident-risk do is to take greater precautions to protect it. But even so, it does not figure more in their thought, and the idea is usually absent that the brain is our workshop and all that we observe, think or imagine happens inside its bony frame.

There are glaring discrepencies in the conventional argument adduced by Underhill. The lyrical mystical ecstasy which attracts and inspires us is comparatively of recent origin, dating at the earliest from a period of not more than three thousand years before the birth of Christ. Before that the picture of religion and the ecstatic trance is more ugly than beautiful. We should not forget the trance of the Shaman, the medicine-man, the witch-doctor and the magi which, too, among their contemporaries betokened ascent to the spirit-world or intercourse with supernatural beings. But often there was hardly any element of the divine or the sublime as we understand it today, in those states of entrancement. The rapture, the clearly marked expansion of self and the sense of identity with all creation, which marked the later expressions of the ecstatic state, are not noticeable in the earlier types, or at least in the remnants of them which survived during historical times. It is a moot issue whether the subjects of those ecstacies were mentally advanced enough even to entertain those feelings as the later mystics did.

There were many gods and goddesses, human, divine or demonic even in the form of animals, birds, reptiles and fish, that demanded bizarre types of worship and ritual, including human sacrifice, cannibalism, self-mutilation, infanticide, obnoxious ceremonies, revolting sexual orgies and the like. It is not wise to overlook, in our zeal to find a supernatural explanation for mystical ecstasy, the dark side of religion or religious experience in the primitive phases of human culture nor the barbarous features that attended the birth and growth of current faiths—forced conversion, ruthless persecution, bloody wars and massacres, pillage and rape, the curse of untouchability, the revolting custom of sati, self-emasculation, the horrors of the Inquisition and the rest.

The mystics, whose writings or recorded histories are before us, do not even form one billionth of the population that lived on earth and passed away during this period. Why they alone were gifted that way we do not know. Why even now hardly one out of myriads reports success in the same endeavor is still an enigma. Millions of aspirants to Samadhi in India abandon their homes, dwell in solitude, practise every form of austerity, penance and self-discipline, meditate and pray day and night without coming anywhere near this state of indescribable beatitude. Were the 'sense' of Timeless Being an integral part of man's spiritual consciousness, as argued by Underhill, then the Vision of Reality would be equally accessible to all, of course, with variations in the degree of success gained, as happens when a class of students attends a university course to widen their knowledge or a group of athletes works in a gymnasium to streamline their bodies. If this view were correct, the 'Vision' would have been the same for the cave dwellers of the neolithic age as it is for the cultured products of this day. But we know this is not the case and the two are poles apart. Why in our religious beliefs do we overlook the past?

The extreme rarity of success in this enterprise has been clearly recognized in India. "Among thousands of men," says the Bhagavad-Gita, "scarce one striveth for perfection, and of the successful strivers, scarce one knoweth me in essence." But even this rare one who achieves the blessed union has, according to the Indian tradition, behind him an accumulated store of meritorious actions done in previous lives, which form the seeds of success in his present one. Explaining this, the Gita says: "But a Yogi, laboring with assiduity, purified from sin, fully perfected through manifold births, he reacheth the supreme goal." This is emphasized again at another place: "At the close of many births, the man full of wisdom cometh unto Me; 'Vasudeva is all'; saith he, the Mahatma very difficult to find."*

It is obvious that the glorious consummation of human life, of which the Gita sings, and of which a glowing picture is presented in the writings of all great mystics of the past, cannot be the work of a day or even of a lifetime, unless there are constitutional factors favorable to the climax, of which we have no knowledge yet. In this respect, the great mystics can be classed with the great secular geniuses of the earth. The mystical consciousness of an Eckhart, or Al-Ghazali or a Chaitanya, is not possible for even one out of hundreds of thousands of earnest practisers of yoga or other spiritual disciplines, in the same way as the intellectual achievement of a Shankara or Einstein is not possible for every scholar or university professor. What these constitutional factors are, it will be my endeavor to explain.

I have briefly touched on the views expressed by Evelyn Underhill, as representative of a religious bent of mind, which believes in God and the divine nature of the Soul. For the views representative of modern psychology, I shall turn to William James and quote him at some length to show the wide divergence in the two points of view. The trouble starts when the Freudian psychologists on the one side, behaviorists on the other, transper-

---

* *Bhagavad-Gita*, 7:19

sonal on the third, anthropologists on the fourth, physicists on the fifth, philosophers on the sixth, theologians on the seventh, the laity on the eighth, the Vedantists on the ninth, the occultists on the tenth and, to crown it all, the mystics themselves on the eleventh, express highly divergent views on the same phenomenon, using all the embellishments of language and the resources of intellect to make their point, without even one calling in for evidence the one single witness of all the happenings in this historically ageless scene. Not one of them even mentions the brain.

"The last aspect of religious life which remains for me to touch upon," writes James, "is the fact that its manifestations so frequently connect themselves with the subconscious part of our existence. You may remember what I said in my opening lecture about the prevalence of the psychopathic temperment in religious biography. You will in point of fact hardly find a religious leader of any kind in whose life there is no record of automatisms. I speak not merely of savage priests and prophets, whose followers regard automatic utterance and action as by itself tantamount to inspiration, I speak of leaders of thought and subjects of intellectualized experience. Saint Paul had his visions, his ecstacies, his gift of tongues, small as was the importance he attached to the latter. The whole array of Christian saints and heresiarchs, including the greatest, the Bernards, the Loyolas, the Luthers, the Foxes, the Wesleys, had their visions, voices, rapt conditions, guiding impressions and 'openings.' They had these things because they had exalted sensibility, and to such things persons of exalted sensibility are liable. In such liability there lie, however, consequences for theology. Beliefs are strengthened wherever automatisms corroborate them. Incursions from beyond the transmarginal region have a peculiar power to increase conviction. The inchoate sense of presence is infinitely stronger than conception, but strong as it may be, it is seldom equal to the evidence of hallucination. Saints who actually see or hear their Saviour reach the acme of assurance. Motor automatism though rarer is, if possible, even more convincing than sensations. The subjects here actually feel themselves played upon by powers beyond their will. The evidence is dynamic; the God or spirit moves the very organs of their body."*

"When, in addition to these phenomena of inspiration," adds William James, "we take religious mysticism into account, when we recall the striking and sudden unification of a discordant self which we saw in conversion, and when we review the extravagant obsessions of tenderness, purity and self-severity met with in saintliness, we cannot, I think, avoid the conclusion that in religion we have a department of human nature with unusually close relations to the transmarginal or subliminal region. If the word 'subliminal' is offensive to any of you, as smelling too much of psychical research or other aberrations, call it by any other name you please, to distinguish it from the level of full sunlit consciousness. Call this latter the A-region of personality, if you care to, and call the other the B-region. The B-region, then, is obviously the larger part of each of us, for it is the abode of everything that is latent and the reservoir of everything that passes unrecorded or unobserved. It contains, for example, such things as all our momentarily inactive memories, and it harbors the springs of all our obscurely motive passions, impulses, likes, dislikes and prejudices. Our intuitions, hypothesies, fancies, superstitions, persuasions, convictions, and in general, all our non-rational operations, come from it. It is the source of our dreams, and apparently they may return to it. In it arise whatever mystical experiences we may have, and our automatisms, sensory or motor; our life in hypnotic and 'hypnoid' conditions, if we are subjects of such conditions; our delusions, fixed ideas, and hysterical accidents, if we are hysteric subjects; our supra-normal cognitions, if such there be, and if we are telepathic subjects. It is also the fountainhead of such that feeds our religion. In persons deep in the religious life, as we have now abundantly seen—and this is my conclusion—the door into this region seems unusually wide open; at any rate,

---

* William James, *The Varieties of Religious Experience*

experiences making their entrance through that door have had emphatic influence in shaping religious history."*.

This is where we land at the end—the bottomless hollow of the unconscious, the sub-conscious, below-the-surface, transmarginal and subliminal mind. This is the hidden region of our personality which, they say, stalks on the stage in dreams, hypnotic and somnambulistic conditions, in hysteria and insanity, in genius and inspiration, in mediumistic displays and extrasensory perception, in possession, obsession and fixations, in cracks, twists and kinks in the brain; in fact, in all the abnormal, paranormal, extraordinary or inexplicable conditions of the mind.

But has anyone explained why in some it leads to nightmares, in some to happy dreams, in some to a mixture of the two and in some to dreamless sleep? Why some are somnambulists, others not; why some are suggestible and others more intractable; why, in some, it leads to the highest purity and nobility of character, as in mystics and, in some, to revolting compulsions or horrible perversions; which make them act more like brutes than human beings; why in some it leads to the horrors of insanity and in some to the joy of creation? What rational solution is this that leaves everything unexplained? To say religion and religious experience come from the unconscious is to shift the venue to another compartment of the same mind. But, whether from this compartment or that, mind is the bastion from which these incursions and invasions, insidious or sudden, come. This we know, but how?

Were we to believe implicitly the saga of the 'unconscious,' the suggestion would be irresistible that we harbour in our interior the arch-fiend himself, and fall victim to his machinations every moment of our lives. He turns into psychopaths the rare few who have the Vision of God, into lunatics the handful who create or discover new treasures for the race, shocks the pure and innocent in dreams or maddens the good and gentle with appalling fear in wakefulness! Where is the man who can truthfully

---

* Ibid

declare that he has subdued this invincible giant? Who has taken a census yet or alleviated the anguish of myriads who watch daily with horror, grief or shock the unpredictable obliquities of their own mind? Does all this cart-load of fears, sorrows and sins rumble out of the cavernous 'unconscious' or does it symbolize a slice of the torment reserved for rebellious man for partaking of the forbidden fruit?

4

Mysticism or Pathology

In dealing with ecstasy, we are face to face with a most profound, constantly repeated phenomenon of religious experience. The real cause for this extraordinary state of mental absorption, attended often by insensibility to the external world and a cataleptic condition of the body, is still unknown. Many among the seekers after self-awareness, ecstasy, sartori, samadhi or God-realization have often no clear-cut idea of the final goal to which the discipline they are undertaking would lead; or that the samadhi brought about by Yoga, the ecstatic trance of the Christian mystics, sartori among the Zen, the state of absorption of the Sufis and the union of Shakti with Shiva of the Tantriks, signify, when genuine, the same experience. But there can be artificially induced or pathological conditions of the mind which present the same external symptoms but lack completely in the subjective elements of the genuine ecstasy.

It is clear that drugs like LSD, mescaline, preparations of opium, hashish, marijuana and the rest in some inexplicable way affect our consciousness. Since these drugs are either taken by mouth or smoked or injected the inference is clear that they affect the blood and the chemistry of the brain in some way which creates a powerful effect on the mind. From this it follows that even our food and drink must be affecting our consciousness, although in a manner which is not perceptible to us except when due to excess or the ingestion of a disagreeable, putrid or poisoned article of food, we feel an adverse reaction both in our body and the mind. The feeling of well-being after a good, wholesome meal and of uneasiness or nausea after an ill-cooked, unsavory or unwholesome one provide an indication of this fact. Any hallucinogen, irritant or excitant consumed by us affects, irritates or excites the brain matter first.

From the way our waking consciousness is affected by the conditon of our blood or what we eat or drink or smoke, it is obvious that the same process must be at work in our dream awareness also, and our bodily or visceral conditions must be reflected in the dreams. We little know what happens to the brain cells by constant fretting, irritation or excitement. But we can make a guess by recalling the smart caused by a caustic or the effects of irritation caused to the skin by a coarse, ill-fitting or very tight article of dress. The analogies can be multiplied. What is important to remember is that our brain is not as immune to abuse, hurt or ill-treatment as we suppose it to be.

In the light of this fact it should be easy to imagine what harm we cause to the grey-matter by excess, vice and violence. But for a prompt repair system, humanity would be a race of maniacs in a few generations only. Most of this repair work is done in the ever-active brain in sleep when we are powerless to interfere! This is the main benefit we derive from the ministrations of our heaven-provided nocturnal nurse.

Many of the current interpretations of dreams are arbitrary and fictitious. There is order and not chaos in our interior. Neither the angel nor the beast runs amok. If there is a fault, it is in ourselves. Our constitution or heredity needs correction. If there is order in atoms and their parts, there cannot be disorder in the ethereal constituents of consciousness. Our dreams hold up a mirror to the surface consciousness to look at herself critically in a manner which, out of vanity and self-love, she never does during the waking hours. They are prophetic, admonitory, reformative, expository or timeless, like mythologies and the inspired material contained in the religious books of various faiths. Our dream scenario can also be an absurd, unintelligible or confused amalgam, depending every time on the state of the neurons. It will take mankind ages to understand the signs.

With this position before our eyes, showing how intimately the body and the mind are interconnected, it is hard to believe that an unprecedented mental state, betokening union with the Almighty and filled with unutterable bliss—never known on the earthly plane—can be the experience of the mind or soul alone, without involving the body or the brain. However brief it might be, the transcendental flight of the soul must be reflected in the cerebral matter in some way. Conversely, it can happen that as the result of a reaction caused in the brain by intense concentration, constant worship, prayer, extreme longing for the beatific vision or consuming love of God, continued for long periods of time, a process of transformation would start in the organ conducive to the extraordinary experiences of the mystical type. The current explanations for astonishing states of mind, as for instance those of child-prodigies, lightning calculators, mediums and mystics, are mostly hypothetical, the result of cogitation by intelligent minds. They are not the fruit of direct experience because the elements involved are too subtle for empirical study. The result is a multi-colored dish of highly spiced cuisine, cooked up by a bright cluster of star mind-healers of our time.

The phenomenon cannot be explained only in theophantic terms, viz. that it represents communion of the soul with God, but also in terms of a revolution caused in the fabric of the brain. The experiences with LSD and mescalin clearly show to what an amazing extent chemical reagents can affect the state of a normal mind. This fact should provide food for reflection not only to the religious-minded, but also to every honest savant engaged in the study of higher consciousness. For the latter, rather than resort to the naive explanation that mystical ecstasy is an exhibit of the subconscious, would it not be more rational to look for a solution to the riddle in the encephalon, if not in the entire organism of the individual. Even if a product of the subconscious, the magnitude of the phenomenon and its impact on the personality make a look at the brain necessary, on the analogy of the study done on genius and insanity.

In the light of the fact that the human organism is a chemical laboratory of a most elaborate kind, the possibility of a bio-chemical synthetic process in the neuronic material to create a different pattern of consciousness, as happens in the case of certain drugs, cannot be ruled out. In fact, there is a growing apperception of the fact that mental disorder can be the immediate result of organic imbalances in the brain. It is to this aspect of Mystical Ecstasy that I wish to draw the attention of the world. Once the study of this rare state of mind is taken up and pursued with vigor, as is done in the other branches of science, a two-fold harvest is sure to result: (1) a clear understanding of the mystical trance, and (2) a widening of the horizon of science itself.

Instead of introducing a supernatural factor or a subterranean cavern in mind itself to account for a historical phenomenon, would it not be more rational to hold that since a distressful, depressive or painful mental condition in an individual can be caused by a disorder of the mind or body, the reverse can also be true and the intensely blissful, elevating and rapturous transport of mystical ecstasy can be the result of a better and more harmonious state of the organic frame. We are not able to decide or even envision this possibility because of the scanty knowledge of our nerves and the brain. How a scientific mind can believe that a psychological fire-work can start in an individual without involving the cerebrum is hard to understand.

The accounts of the mystics are so varied and their experiences so paradoxical and so diverse in character—a compound of exaltation and depression, ecstasy and agony, hope and despair, light and darkness—so influenced by the state of health, age, mental disposition and environment of the subjects that, in its external features the phenomenon is no different from the other psychological states of human beings. Were mystical ecstasy only a spirit to spirit encounter with incorporeal Divinity, the bodily or mental state of the mystic would not be allowed to color the experience. But this is not the case. On the contrary, the stress and strain caused on the system of a contemplative—entrancement, contortion of the body, epileptic seizure, diminished pulse and breathing, hysteria and, sometimes, even convulsion—tell a different tale. Correctly understood, in the light of studies already done, mystical ecstasy is a psychosomatic phenomenon which can be investigated if approached in the right way.

The views expressed by Underhill and other able writers on mysticism, as also the avowals made by mystics themselves, make it clear beyond doubt that in the genuine mystical trance the subject loses, wholly or partially, the awareness of the world and experiences a state of lucidity and self-expansion in which the soul apprehends its oneness with God or a Divine Imminence, variously delineated, attended by a rapture which is unique. The artificially induced states resulting from certain passive types of meditation, arrest of breathing, Khechari mudra, repetition of sounds, gazing at bright objects or the tip of the nose, or other methods of self-hypnosis, used by some well-known mystics too, as for instance Boehme, though alike in external symbology, do not betoken genuine ecstasy and often lead to serious error in evaluating the true condition.

Commenting on this aspect of the mystical trance, Underhill writes: "There are three distinct aspects under which the ecstatic state may be studied: (a) the physical, (b) psychological, (c) the mystical. Many of the deplorable misunderstandings and still more deplorable mutual recriminations, which surround its discussion, come from the refusal of experts in one of these three branches to consider the results arrived at by the other two. Physically considered, ecstasy is a trance; more or less deep, more or less prolonged. The subject may slide into it gradually from a period of absorption in, or contemplation of, some idea which has filled the field of consciousness; or, it may come on suddenly, the appearance of the idea—or even some word or symbol suggesting the idea—abruptly throwing the subject into an entranced condition. This is the state which some mystical writers call rapture. The distinction, however, is a conventional one and the works of the mystics describe many intermediate forms.

"During the trance, breathing and circulation are depressed. The body is more or less cold or rigid, remaining in the exact position which it occupied at the oncoming of the ecstasy, however difficult and unnatural this pose may be. Sometimes entrancement is so deep there is complete anaesthesia, as in the case which I quote from the life of St. Catherine of Siena. Credible witnesses report that Bernadette, the visionary of Lourdes, held the flaming end of a candle in her hand for fifteen minutes during one of her ecstasies. She felt no pain, neither did the flesh show any marks of burning. Similar instances of ecstatic anaesthesia abound in the lives of the saints, and are also characteristic of certain pathological states."*

"The mystics themselves are fully aware of the importance of this distinction," continues Underhill. "Ecstasies, no less than visions and voices must, they declare, be subjected to unsparing criticism before they are recognized as divine: whilst some are undoubtedly 'of God,' others are no less clearly 'of the devil.' 'The great doctors of the mystic life,' says Malaval, 'teach that there are two sorts of rapture, which must be carefully distinguished. The first are produced in persons but little advanced in the Way, and still full of selfhood; either by the force of a heated imagination which vividly apprehends a sensible object, or by the artifice of the devil. These are the raptures which St. Teresa calls, in various parts of her works, Raptures of Feminine Weakness. The other sort of Rapture is, on the contrary, the effect of pure intellectual vision in those who have a great and generous love for God. To generous souls who have utterly renounced themselves, God never fails in these raptures to communicate high things.' "

"Sometimes both kinds of ecstasy, the healthy and the psychopathic," adds Underhill, "are seen in the same person. Thus in the

---

* Evelyn Underhill, *Mysticism*

cases of St. Catherine of Genoa and St. Catherine of Siena it would seem that as their health became feebler and the nervous instability always found in persons of genius increased, the ecstasies became more frequent; but they were not healthy ecstasies, such as those which they experienced in the earlier stages of their careers, and which brought with them an excess of vitality. They were the result of increasing weakness of the body, not of the over-powering strength of the spirit: and there is evidence that Catherine of Genoa, that acute self-critic, was conscious of this. Those who attended on her did not know how to distinguish one state from the other. And hence on coming to, she would sometimes say, 'Why did you let me remain in this quietude, from which I have almost died?' "*

I have again cited Evelyn Underhill at some length as it is needless to recapitulate what has been said on this point by a well-known sympathetic writer on mysticism. What does this study reveal? Does it not show that mystical ecstasy is not an experience of the spirit alone, but that the body, nervous system and the brain of the mystic are inextricably interwoven with it? Assuming for the sake of argument that the audience of the soul with God causes such an impact on the corporeal sheath that by the sheer force of it all the vitality in the body is drawn up and it lies motionless in a swoon, insensible to itself and the world around for the period of the communion, the position still remains that the embodied spirit, in her encounter with the Divine, cannot leave the corpus behind but, whether fainting or conscious, inert or active, has to carry it along with herself whenever the audience takes place. Since the spirit is herself a ray or spark of the Divine, it is evident that if the corporeal form develops the capacity to bear the Splendor, manifested at the time of the intercourse, the meeting or the union can be possible any and every time. This is what I have in mind when I refer to further evolution of the brain. This is what Yoga and other spiritual disciplines are designed for.

---

* Ibid

What more evidence is needed to show that the body and the brain play a signal role in bringing about the mystical trance than the avowals of some mystics themselves that ecstasies, visions and voices should be subjected to closest scrutiny, before they are accepted as divine, for some of them are undoubtedly of God and others no less clearly of the devil. If this interpretation of chaste and unchaste ecstasies is literally accepted, it would mean putting the whole subject of mystical vision in serious uncertainty and doubt. This can make one suspicious of the genuine experience as well, for in supporting such a point of view, we regress to the primitive superstitious belief that what is good comes from God and what is evil from the arch-enemy of man. To an unbiased mind, it should be palpably clear that a rational explanation for the polarity in the two ecstasies can only be that in one case the organism is well-adjusted for the experience. In the second, it is not. It is the state of preparedness of the percipients' brain that makes the ecstasy beneficient and divine in one case or malefi-cient and diabolical in the other. The same individual can have both types, at different times, corresponding to the condition of the brain.

There is still a serious misunderstanding about the real nature of the mystical trance. I say serious because the consequences of this ignorance about a phenomenon of great historical impor-tance, as the seed-bed of all the four current major faiths of man-kind, with all the eventualities which emerged from them during the past two thousand years, and still continue to emerge, can prove distressful for the race. This is not all. It will, perhaps, never become known how many hundreds of thousand souls, thirsting for self-knowledge, during the last few decades, unable to resist the urge and, at the same time, in confusion about the real nature of their thirst on account of the chaos existing in this province, went from pillar to post and from post to pillar in their search, to fall victim to deception, drugs, disease and degeneration for lack of correct knowledge of and right guidance on the path. When the scores are reckoned, on whom will fall the responsibility for this default?

"It need hardly be said," adds Underhill, "that rationalistic writers, ignoring the parallels offered by the artistic and philosophic temperments, have seized eagerly upon the evidence afforded by such instances of apparent mono-ideism and self hypnotization in the lives of the mystics, and by the physical disturbances which accompany the ecstatic trance, and sought by its application to attribute all the abnormal perceptions of contemplative genius to hysteria or other disease. They have not hesitated to call St. Paul an epileptic, St. Teresa the 'patron saint of hysterics;' and have found room for most of their spiritual kindred in various departments of the pathological museum. They have been helped in this grateful task by the acknowledged fact that the great contemplatives, though almost always persons of robust intelligence and marked practical or intellectual ability—Plotinus, St. Bernard, the two St. Catherines, St. Teresa, St. John of the Cross, and the Sufi poets Jami and Jalalu 'ddin are cases in point—have often suffered from bad physical health. More, their mystical activities have generally reacted upon their bodies in a definite and special way; producing in several cases a particular kind of illness and of physical disability, accompanied by pains and functional disturbances for which no organic cause could be discovered, unless that cause were the immense strain which exalted spirit puts upon a body which is adapted to a very different form of life."*

In the concluding portion of the paragraph, Underhill comes nearer to the truth than, perhaps, she herself suspected. It is "the immense strain caused on the body by an exalted spirit" which is at the bottom of the degenerative tendencies and pathological conditions associated not only with the mystical personality, but, more pointedly, with genius also. Considered in the light of the fact that mental abberation, eccentricity, neurosis and insanity have been a common feature of exceptionally gifted minds, instead of a sweeping generalization that genius is a form of insanity, and collection of voluminous data to support this view, would it not

---

* Ibid

have been more rational to concede that the reason for this peculiarity could lie in the excessive consumption of psychic energy by a mind more brilliant, more fertile, more artistic or more imaginative than an average one? It is ignorance about the working of the brain and the energy nourishing it which is at the base of the highly mistaken notions current about genius or that form of it which manifests itself in the mystical mind.

"The progress of science," says Whitehead, "consists in observing and in showing with a patient ingenuity that the events of this ever-shifting work are but examples of a few general connections or relations called laws. To see what is general in what is particular and what is permanent in what is transitory is the aim of scientific thought. In the eye of science, the fall of an apple, the motion of a planet around a sun, and the clinging of the atmosphere to the earth are all seen as examples of the law of gravity. This possibility of disentangling the most complex evanescent circumstances into various examples of permanent laws is the controlling idea of modern thought."* We are not able to disentangle the highly complex problems, presented by genius, mystical ecstasy and psychosis because bewildered by the diversity of the features, peculiar to each, we fail to detect the single thread that runs through all of them due to the habit of our isolating thought from the brain.

Underhill's criticism of the views expressed by rationalist writers is not well-timed. The provocation is from the other side. If someone claims that he had intercourse with the Almighty and, instead of providing incontestable evidence in support of it, comes off from the encounter with a sickly body and a schizoid mind, the doubt created would be fully justified. In fact, those who are confident of their theistic interpretation of the experience should be all too ready to satisfy the doubts. Scholars have been unsparing in their views about geniuses, exposing ruthlessly their mental and physical faults, although most of them never

---

* Whitehead, *Introduction to Mathematics*

claimed special divine favor. So there appears to be no reason why mystics should be treated differently in those cases where there is a similar or even greater departure from normalcy. In this context, the view expressed by William James, another well-known authority on religious experiences, is worthy of note:

"The classic religious mysticism, it now must be confessed," says James, "is only a privileged case.' It is an extract, kept true to type by the selection of the fittest specimens and their preservation in 'schools.' It is carved out from a much larger mass; and if we take the larger mass as seriously as religious mysticism has taken itself, we find historically that the supposed unanimity largely disappears. To begin with, even religious mysticism itself, the kind that accumulates traditions and makes schools, is much less unanimous than I have allowed. It has been both ascetic and antinominally self-indulgent within the Christian church. It is dualistic in Sankhya, and monistic in Vedanta philosophy. I called it pantheistic; but the great Spanish mystics are anything but pantheists. They are with few exceptions non-metaphysical minds, for whom 'the category of personality' is absolute. The 'union' of man with God is for them much more like an occasional miracle than like an original identity."

"How different again, apart from the happiness common to all," continues William James, "is the mysticism of Walt Whitman, Edward Carpenter, Richard Jeffries and other naturalistic pantheists, from the more distinctively Christian sort. The fact is that mystical feeling of enlargement, union and emancipation has no specific intellectual content whatever of its own. It is capable of forming matrimonial alliances with materials furnished by the most diverse philosophies and theologies, provided only they can find a place in their framework for its peculiar emotional mood. We have no right, therefore, to invoke its prestige as distinctively in favor of any special belief, such as that in absolute idealism, or in the absolute monistic identity, or in the absolute goodness of the world. It is only relatively in favor of all these things—it passes out of common human consciousness in the direction in which they lie."*

"So much for religious mysticism proper. But more remains to be told, for religious mysticism is only one half of mysticism. The other half has no accumulated traditions accept those which the text books on insanity supply. Open any one of these and you will find abundant cases in which 'mystical ideas' are cited as characteristic symptoms of enfeebled or deluded states of mind. In delusional insanity, paranoia, as they sometimes call it, we may have a diabolical mysticism, a sort of religious mysticism turned upside down. The same sense of ineffable importance in the smallest events, the same texts and words coming with new meanings, the same voices and visions and leadings and missions, the same controlling by extraneous powers; only this time the emotion is pessimistic: instead of consolation we have desolation; the meanings are dreadful; and the powers are enemies to life. It is evident that from the point of view of their psychological mechanism, the classic mysticism and these lower mysticisms spring from the same mental level, from the great subliminal or transmarginal region of which science is beginning to admit the existence, but of which so little is really known. That region contains every kind of matter; 'seraph and snake' abide there side by side. To come from thence is no infallible credential. What comes must be sifted and tested, and run the gauntlet of confrontation with the total context of experience, just like what comes from the outer world of sense. Its value must be ascertained by empirical methods, so long as we are not mystics ourselves."*

The aim of knowledge is to throw light on what is obscure, to explain what is inexplicable and to solve what is problematic. We cannot call that knowledge which makes the obscure darker, the inexplicable even more so and the enigmatic more perplexing than before. Nor is that knowledge which, instead of answering a riddle, explains it by another even harder than the one answered by it. This is the position adopted by modern psychology in deal-

---

* William James, *The Varieties of Religious Experience*
* Ibid

ing with the abnormal and paranormal phenomena of the mind. Other than this how can we classify the attempt made to explain psychosis, automatism, inspiration, mystical ecstasy or extra-sensory perception in terms of the 'unconscious,' an entity more puzzling, more mysterious and more foreign to us than the phenomena which they try to explain by it.

We can no more divide the mind into conscious and uncons-cious parts than we can divide the flowing water gliding down the sandy bed of a winding river. We can only see the upper surface of the current, its ripples, waves, whirlpools and eddies and not the, by far, larger mass of water gliding below, hidden by the upper layer from our sight. For this, we do not make a distinction between the top and the bottom levels of water, but call the whole mass a river, not the 'surface river' and the 'under-the-surface river.' In fact, it would be a mistake to do so as there is a constant inter-change of water between the upper and lower layers of the current; water from the surface coming down and that under it rising up in a swirling motion, as the river flows on.

Like a measureless, all-encompassing river, the stream of con-sciousness flows on day and night. Its ripples, waves, whirlpools and eddies represent the revolutions, upheavals and cataclysmic ups and downs of life. A river rises from the waters of the ocean as nebulous vapor condensing into a very fine atomized spray that gathers into drops, descending on the earth as rain, hail or snow, to form into a stream which flows on and on until its water mingles again with the ocean wherefrom it had come. It is one. Its division into two parts, the 'upper' and the 'lower' is unrealistic as the water is in movement up and down everywhere.

Mind has a cosmic dimension in which our individual minds are like drops of water in an ocean or extremely slender beams of light radiating from a gigantic sun. Our mind knows all about us for it is the intelligence in us while we know only as much as we are permitted to do, according to the capacity of the brain. How it has been assumed that each individual mind is restricted to one par-ticular body, in two divisions, the upper and the lower, is a riddle. Can highly rarified mediums, like ether and light, or gases like hydrogen, helium and air or even liquids like water, spirit or oil, be separated into parts or prevented from spreading out without the use of impervious containers or the erection of impenetrable partition walls?

How then can it be supposed that mind, subtler than all of them, can stay in isolated units, clinging to the highly porous mortal frame of each living creature, without intermingling with the surrounding fields? The position remains unaffected whether mind is considered to be a chance product of organic activity or as a self-existing constituent of the Universe. It also remains unaffected whether it is held to be incorporeal, etheric or organic in its composition.

Why I wish to draw attention to this obvious fact is because the current concepts of psychology about mind debase and disfigure the holy image of consciousness, the sublime object of man's eternal quest. This error in thinking is the outcome of an incorrect approach to the study of mind and insufficient knowledge of the brain. When even the physicists have been driven to admit that, at its finest levels, matter is becoming more and more difficult to explore and the behavior of its elementary particles harder and harder to determine, how can the dogmatic premises of psychology about an element, inaccessible to sensory observation and by far more subtle and complex than the former be accepted as correct? I am constrained to point this out because in its existing form and with its present methods of investigation, the current science of mind, by denigrating the high ideals and supernal beliefs of religion, is doing more harm than good to the race.

If a distinction is to be made it would be more appropriate to call one 'incarnate' and the other 'discarnate' mind. This, too, is only a man-made distinction for the drop is never out of the ocean and the rays of light never cut off from the sun. There is no 'unconscious' mind. The very idea is a contradiction in terms. The areas, further away from our awareness, are as highly conscious and intelligent as the rest and even more so. It is, as it were, a plumbless ocean of intelligence everywhere. The fantasies of childhood, the traumatic experiences of puberty and the savage traits of our remote ancestors cling to us—the drops of the always unsullied waters of the ocean—as a result of contaminations arising from embodiment.

The water of the river carries various kinds of matter held in suspension which makes it muddy and impure. It is these impurities which lend a particular tint, taste or even odor to the fluid. Cleared of them it is uniformly pure, both in its upper and lower reaches. The floating sediment, because of its heaviness, gravitates towards the bottom and finally settles down as silt on the bed and the banks of the river. When interwoven with the body, our mind too, carries impurities in suspension which gravitate more toward the lower reaches, closer to the flesh. Otherwise, this ethereal stuff is perenially stainless and pure.

It is the more or less purity of this marvellous element of creation in the embodied form which determines our daily cheerful and heavy moods, the delightful or unpleasant contents of our dream scenes at night, the fertile and barren periods of genius, the delirious and lucid intervals or manic and depressive phases of insanity and the enrapturing flights to heaven or gloomy descents into hell of the mystical mind. It is these impurities which cause the psychopathic syndrome in countless minds living on the borderline of sanity—abnormal behavior, sexual perversion, obsession, possession, uncontrollable impulses, urges, appetites and the rest. The more a mind is sensitive, penetrating and intelligent, the more likelihood there is of its susceptibility to psychic ills. There are impurities and toxins in the nerves and the brain as there are viruses and poisons in the blood and other tissues of the body. But the subtle nerve and brain poisons are of a different kind. They will be amenable to control, when once sufficient insight is gained into this still obscure parameter of organic life.

The modern psychologist sits on the horns of a dilemma. He must preserve his peace with the anthropologist and the biologist. At the same time, he must not stray too far from the prevalent orthodox ideas and beliefs on which he is brought up and bred in the university. It is hard to be a rebel and run the gauntlet of a host, or forego the 'hurrah' of appreciative colleagues on one's performance. Otherwise, it should not be difficult for an intelligent student of mind to realize that the subject under his study is bristling with contradictions and unsolved problems. There is more of make-believe material in his books than of real insight into the phenomena. For this reason, instead of focusing his attention at the spot where the unearthed secrets of this element of nature lie buried deep in the soil of the body, he is compelled to wander here and there in search of them. The following words of Jung ring as true today as they did in his time.

"There is not one modern psychology," he says, "there are dozens of them. This is curious enough when we remember that there is only one science of mathematics, of geology, zoology, botany and so forth. But there are so many psychologies that an American university was able to publish a thick volume under the title, *Psychologies of 1930.* I believe there are as many psychologies as philosophies, for there is also no single philosophy but many. I mention this for the reason that philosophy and psychology are linked by indissoluable bonds which are kept in being by the inter-relation of their subject-matters. Psychology takes the psyche for its subject, and philosophy—to put it briefly—takes the world."* When there are so many psychologies that a directory becomes necessary, where is a person with a pressing psychological problem sitting heavy on his mind to go in order to find a correct solution for it?

The basic features of consecrated religious life have always been the same—unwavering belief in a higher power, truthfulness, fellow-feeling, purity of heart, compassion and a passionate desire for self-conquest. Wherever we look, a mosaic of these traits is found to be a common characteristic of the enlightened mind in any part of the earth. How could a phenomenon so widespread in space, so extended in time and so rich in the wealth of ideals and principles be brushed aside in the search for knowledge

---

* C.G. Jung, *Psychological Reflections* edited by J. Jacobi

in recent times? The responsibility of this rather strange behavior is shared both by religion and science—by the former on account of its dogmatic insistence on the infallibility of Revelation and the latter for the same over-emphasis on the infallibility of the intellect!

The fact that mind is incorporeal and cosmic does not affect the position that, in some way unknown to us, it can affect material forces or particles and, in turn, be influenced by them. Without this action and reaction embodied life, as we know it, would not be possible. We cannot refuse to determine this relationship between mind and cerebral matter on the ground that the objective world, in which the human body and the brain are included, are but illusory creations of this universal mind. To assume this would be to put an end to the progress of knowledge and even of embodied mind itself. The assumption that all we see around is a product of consciousness is a greater reason why we should redouble our efforts at finding answers to the riddles encountered. This assumption would naturally include what we think, imagine, do or plan as also the riddles we encounter and the efforts we make to solve them, are all the ingredients of this illusory display. That being the case, common sense demands that the rules of the same be applied to all the constituents of this illusion and not only to some. This means that they apply also to the relationship between the mind and the brain.

If it is supposed that mind is the product of material elements at their primary levels, that is at the level of atoms or even below, in that case, too, it will have to be admitted that this extremely subtle or complex biochemical product must in some way be interwoven or interconnected with neurons and act on the body in a manner unintelligible to us at this time. In either case, in order to solve the mystery, there can be no denying of the fact that brain is the most likely place where we can look for a solution to the problem presented by the mind.

The examination of a dissected brain, or the data transmitted by an electro-encephalograph or knowledge of the chemical composition of neurons, or study of sleep or insanity or of yogis cannot yield to us any specific information about the nature of the mind or its relationship to the brain, for the simple reason that the element involved is too subtle, too intricate and too inextricably interconnected with cerebral and nerve substances to become a separate object of empirical investigation, as is the case with materials and forces with which science has been dealing so far. The presumption that mind, or the stuff of which our thoughts and feelings are made, does not possess any property by which it can become perceptible to our senses, can only lead to the conclusion that our own mystery would always remain beyond the reach of science.

For this purpose, the first issue to be decided is to determine whether the current methods of empirical study can be applied to an entity which is impervious to sensory perception and utterly devoid of any attribute by which it can be empirically measured or sized. What course then is left for a fair-minded empiricist to reach to the bottom of this mystery? If scientific study of the nature followed in the case of material objects is ruled out, then the only other alternative left is an internal study of the experimenter's own mind, both in its conscious and unconscious contents. The question is: did any empiricist during the last, let us say, two hundred years undertake a self-study of this kind? If no study of this nature was undertaken, we cannot then expect anything better than what has been achieved in the field of psychology so far. It is not for the lover of religion to intercede with the empiricist in this behalf, but it is for the latter to decide whether his own demarcation between the objective world and the spirit is correct.

We have still to grasp the colossal mystery surrounding our existence. Just as by constant attention to and study of the external world we were able to make the amazing progress in the knowledge of matter, of which the fruits are before our eyes, in the same manner by constant attention to and study of the inner world we can make progress in the knowledge of the spirit of which, too, the rich harvest will be no less commensurate with the effort made. But this effort has not been made so far except in the field of religion under an individualistic premise and belief. What is needed is a reverent, impersonal approach to this colossal, super-mundane mystery.

It cannot be said that raw material, as provided by alchemy, astrology, healing arts and natural sciences of olden times, for the physical sciences of today, was not available for the pioneers of the science of mind. It was and, perhaps, is a more lavish measure than for any other branch of knowledge. A huge library of self-revelations and writings of hundreds of earlier luminaries of this branch of knowledge, including among them some of the loftiest figures in history, and a large proportion of the most truthful and honest souls ever born, was right in front of them and only needed the labor of reading to know that a method did exist by which mind could be studied in a far better way than any used by science so far. This galaxy of empiricists of the mind included in its ranks some of the most illustrious figures of the ancient world, from Egypt, China, India, Europe, Arabia, Persia, Japan and other places, whose names are household words even today. They do not belong to one race, one period of time or one creed, but their distinguished array, which stretches to the remotest periods of history, includes all racial types and covers all the faiths of mankind.

It is unbelievable that any disciplined body of truly enlightened intellects could dismiss with but one stroke of the pen the accumulated experience and knowledge of a subject of study, religion in this case, contributed by over two hundred generations of keen observers, some of them tallest in mental acumen and moral stature, as was done by some luminaries of science, during the last two centuries in a manner as if all this reverently preserved material had emanated from an assembly of petty, hare-brained creatures, unworthy of the least notice from the cream of the intelligentsia of our time. The mistake occurred because religion, mystical ecstasy, psychic phenomena, miracles, occultation, alchemy and the rest were viewed in isolation from each other and not as ramifications of an extraordinary activity of the brain, witnessed from a period long before the pyramids were built.

From the time over fifteen hundred years before Moses, in Egypt, to Ramakrishna and Gandhi in India, a span of not less than five thousand years, this special class of human beings has repeated the same story, displayed the same traits of character and followed the same simple pattern of life. How fallible is the human intellect, and how inconstant is the nature of man is demonstrated by the fact that a hundred times more regard was shown, more attention paid, more time and resources spent and more labor done to provide evidence for the guess-work of a nineteenth century naturalist on the Origin of Man, which time is disproving now, than on the study of a recurrent phenomenon relating to the same issue, vouched for by the brightest stars of the firmament of human thought, hundreds in number, covering the whole span of history. How would it reflect, in the days ahead, on the mentality of this rational age when it is decisively proved, on the testimony of the brain, that their collective stand was right and the wild conjecture, aimed to disprove that, grievously wrong? What has prevented the modern giants of learning and the pillars of science from looking more closely into such a prominent and promising field of enquiry, it is hard to say. But, if one is permitted to make a guess, it could be the intoxication of material triumphs, unwarranted prejudice and pride.

5

The Panorama of
Creation

My life has been a fairytale. There have been so many unexpected events and breathtaking incidents that volumes would be needed to recount them. These narratives will appear in the succeeding parts of my autobiography. I have remained a humble, obscure person all my life, my hands full with domestic responsibilities and humane social tasks. I voluntarily took up the latter under the gentle pressure of an urge that I should not live only for myself, but devote at least a fraction of my time to the service of those stricken by misfortune, disability or want, who expect their fellow beings to come to their help, as all of us do in adversity.

The experience I had in 1937 accentuated this urge and finally made me devote a part of the time I could spare to humanitarian work. Sometimes I have a feeling that I survived the ordeal and was able to retain my sanity and my life because my mind remained occupied, for a good part of the day, with the problems of others which prevented it from dwelling obsessively on what was happening in my own interior. There are some who feel agitated when they come across scenes of misery in other people. There are some in whom the feeling is less pronounced and some in whom it is absent altogether. Many among the first group perform little acts of charity and compassion not as a service to others but as a duty owed, not as a meritorious performance but as a measure to relieve the pain they feel at the sight of suffering in a fellow being. It is people of this disposition of whom I have met quite a few in my life whose example I tried to emulate.

It will not be possible for me, even if I write a dozen volumes, to narrate in detail the highly exciting and adventurous life that I lived within. From December, 1937, I have been the dumb spectator of a drama which staged a new act every day. After every few years, the panorama in my interior changed and I found myself in a new world each time with its own allurements and its own problems. It is hard to imagine in what a marvellous country I dwell in my mind. A fairyland would be a poor analogy. The most beautiful palace on earth with mirrors, crystals and gems, everywhere reflecting the milky lustre of hundreds of flourescent lights would be a weak simile to portray the splendorous Eden in which I live and breathe. The frailties of the body, the stresses of the mind, illness, irregularity and, above all, lack of the environment needed for the full bloom of this sublime inner state, at times, undo the enrapturing loveliness of this paradise, like a storm disrupting a festive carnival in a blooming garden, scattering the blossoms and dispersing the holiday crowds in all directions.

I live in a world which is beyond the conception of the most imaginative writer and erudite scholar of our day. I live in a world which is denied to most heads of nations, leaders of thought, commanders of armies, dignitaries of the church, champion athletes, star actors and magnates of trade. I am making these comparisons without the least sense of superiority or the slightest tinge of pride. In fact, nothing can humble one's vanity more than a glimpse of the resplendent world of life. But since, from my point of view, attainment of this state of inner illumination is the immediate target in front of every human being, it is necessary for me to present a true picture of it to the world of assessment. In order to do so, the contrast existing between this sovereign state of inner being and the highest worldly positions, the attainment whereof consumes all the time and bodily resources of the aspirants is necessary to be made.

The profound significance of Viveka—discrimination between what is true and what is false, and Vairagya, a sense of detachment from the world—two of the main pillars on which spiritual discipline is based in India, can be readily grasped in the context of the by far richer harvest of the spiritual quest. Subdual of earthly ambition and passion is necessary to win the far more precious prize of illuminated consciousness. The comparison is necessary to make it clear that the inner kingdom to which man is an heir, surpasses anything which fires the imagination or excites the ambition of human beings. It is a treasure that has no parallel on the earth. Every great mystic of the past came as a divine messenger to draw attention to this glorious consummation in order to make the race aware of her destiny.

What I say now has been said hundreds of times during the last three thousand years. The only difference is that I am repeating the message in a language appropriate to this age. The man of the future will dwell on the earth as we do, with subdued ambition, passion and desire, but with a mind roaming the glowing vault of heaven in ceaseless wonder and ecstasy, his eyes opened to other planes of creation, motivated by other dreams and ambitions and invested with other powers and potentialities than those dreamed of or sought after by us at present.

I have not the least fear that I would be disbelieved or misunderstood or even ridiculed for my outspoken statements. I know what I claim is beyond belief, that no one has narrated a story similar to mine before, nor has the world heard of an adventure parallel to the one I am talking about. From my point of view, mystical ecstasy does not denote an encounter with the Creator, but the birth of a new pattern of consciousness, the common heritage of future man. I have the highest veneration for the mystics of every land and clime. With tears in my eyes, I read of their trials and triumphs, of their sacrifices and the rewards they won, of the pain they endured and the happiness they gained.

It is a privilege for me to count myself as a footman in this august assembly. I have not the least doubt in my mind that the experience is similar, but the interpretation is not. Nor did all of them believe that they had experienced God in this state of enlightenment. Buddha is a notable exception. So are Mahavira and Kapila in India. The interpretation placed by Eckhart or Boehme, on the one side, and St. Francis on the other is not the same. Some held the pantheistic, some theistic and some dualistic views. The same has been the case in Persia, Arabia and India. But all of them are emphatic on the point that the encounter was divine and what they perceived reflected the glory of an Intelligence above that met on the earth.

I do not believe it is possible for the human mind to apprehend the Almighty Creator of the Universe. In order to attain such a power of apprehension, the human mind must first itself rise to that state of cognition. In other words, it must be able to perceive the stupendous Universe in its totality before it can hope to have a correct and intimate knowledge of its Almighty Lord. Can we believe that a droplet of spray, bouncing off the crest of a racing wave, can apprehend the ocean or a whirling grain of sand measure the extent of the Sahara?

The only way in which it can be said that the Almighty can be experienced by the puny human mind is to assume that His glory is spread everywhere and that, in the mystical trance, this glory is perceived much more clearly than in normal consciousness. This is what actually happens. But this does not bespeak a direct encounter with the Source of All—the support behind the Universe and the Light behind the galaxies and stars. In fact, it is only in the degree of perception of this glory, reflected in consciousness or, in other words, in a wider awareness of the world of consciousness that the mystic excels the average human being.

This is where the cerebral cortex comes in. This is the issue which the experiments done would decide. On the verdict of this experiment the fate of the current theories about the origin of man, too, will depend. Those who claimed a real encounter with God in all probability perceived the image already present in their mind, seen in the glow of an expanded consciousness. The transition from normal to transcendental awareness can be so staggering and the state of cognition can attain such a breath-taking proportion that the ego, completely eclipsed and dwarfed, is driven to the conclusion that it is in the presence of an all-pervading Intelligence that can only belong to a super-human Being. The now highly vivified imagination presents the idea in the form of a palpable reality, clothed in glory, majestic in proportion and regal in appearance, corresponding to the new effulgent, highly expanded and sovereign consciousness of the percipient of the Vision himself.

I am presenting this interpretation, not with the aim that it may be accepted without verification, but with the idea that it can provide an alternative explanation for the phenomena of religion and throw a flood of light on the obscurities and anomalies existing in the sacred lore of various faiths, hard to explain in the context of the assumption that the message contained is a direct communication from God. From what I have experienced it is clear that there are other channels of knowledge possible for man which come into operation in transcendental consciousness. Since the experience is so staggering, it is not surprising that the knowledge received in this sublime condition is ascribed to a heavenly Source.

I became convinced about the authenticity of my own experience after a day to day observation extending to many years and, as the outcome of the assurance felt, I published an account of it in the year 1967. It was my hope that the extraordinary nature of the event and the fact that it provided a plausible solution to a host of problems relating to mind, there would be a warm response to it, especially from those interested in the study of mind and consciousness. A good proportion of the readers in many parts of the earth, including scholars of eminence, did become interested in my story. But for reasons which I have still not been able to locate, the idea of an experiment to prove the correctness of my observations did not evoke as enthusiastic a response as could have been expected.

Because of the novelty of the adventure, the press, too, did not show any particular interest in the ideas propounded. I had the first realization of this fact in West Germany. The interviews arranged with press correspondents by my friends proved a failure. They looked at me blankly when I narrated my story and, after a few questions, gave up the task as hopeless. I was saying something they had never heard before and they could not make head or tail of it. Some of them might have even doubted my veracity and some ascribed what I said to the strange notions of an oriental. A correspondent in Philadelphia published a rather amusing version of what I said to him, supported by a photograph as uncomplimentary as the version itself.

If I had walked barefoot over a bed of glowing embers, swiftly for a short distance, or performed a few clever sleights-of-hand before a simple audience under the pretense that I possessed paranormal powers, the news, with a little pulling of strings here and there, would have travelled around the world. Or if I had related the story of an encounter with Yeti, the snowman, or a brush with some other prehistoric monster or some notorious terrorist or a twin of Jack-the-Ripper, the narrative would have been eagerly sought after and avidly read. Or if with a doctorate in science, I had said something fantastic or funny about genetic engineering, still only a doubtful proposition, or about a new exciting wonder in the sky millions of light years away, the statement, with shrieking headlines, would have been before the eyes of millions of readers soon after. Or had a political doyen, even one known for his abberations, supported my stories, the news would have been given prominence by the press, not because they were interested in it, but because a celebrity had endorsed what I said.

But, when I say that the human brain, the most precious possession of every man, woman and child on earth, is in a state of organic transformation, carrying the entire race towards a glorious destination, the news reporters and even the learned cool off, not because the information is not of importance, but because they have never heard of it before. They become disinterested because it seems to them at first sight that the practical side of the idea, even if accepted, is far less than that provided by a better knowledge of the planet Saturn's intriguing system of rings. It seems to them that the excavation of a fossil of a prehistoric animal, extinct some millions of years ago, or the controversial discovery of the lone survivor of an extinct species of whale-like creatures, which often take the academies and the media by storm, is of far more consequence for the race than the fate of her own brain. A worn-out rut that opens out on a rubbish pile is, sometimes, more acceptable to conservative minds than a freshly blazed trail leading to a heap of ambergris.

This is how the world reacted to new discoveries when there were no newspapers and learning was confined only to a few. True to habit, it is reacting in the same way now, when the media cover the earth and academies abound everywhere. To expect instant acceptance of honest truth, unless promoted by a celebrity or peppered with exciting tales, or propelled by a push from wealth or proclaimed by a thousand tongues is to expect the impossible. There is no chance for a lone dreamer, who waits for his truth to triumph on its own merits, to succeed. The erudite, always occupied with intellectual pursuits, have no time to listen to one not adorned with an insignia like theirs, and the press, busy in telling the rosary of notorious Toms and famous Dicks all day, has no place for a commoner. Man is still a slave to wealth, rank and name. Comraderie and equality are but pleasing names.

For me obscurity was, perhaps, a blessing in disguise as it allowed me ample time to study myself and to reflect calmly on the implications of my experience. Limelight, while I was still struggling for clarity, could have dazzled my eyes and turned my head, as it often does in the case of darlings of the media. But I cannot help feeling that there are myriads more worthy of attention from the wardens of publicity, whose sagas of greatness and goodness remain hidden from the world, in contrast to the favorites on whom the media dance attendance every day.

The obsessive fondness of the media for the singular, the bizarre, the frightful, the thrilling and the exciting to make their wares attractive, creates a corresponding excessive craving for the startling, the shocking, the horrifying and the sensational in the readers. When daily indulged in, the craving can assume the proportion of a phobia, extremely harmful for the brain. The feverish eagerness for listening to or reading the news or viewing television and the restlessness often felt, when this is denied, provide an indication to show the abrasion caused on the cortical sheaths. Since the topic is very relevant to our theme, a few words are necessary to show how the present neglect of our headpiece might prove to be the one single factor which can undo all that has been achieved by mankind during recent centuries. Are not most of us assiduously taught from our very childhood how to take care of our teeth, eyes, hair, nails, skin, body, digestion, elimination and the rest. But are we ever instructed in the way we should take care of the very Tree of our life—the brain. For this one omission the present civilization faces a fall!

Where is the sanity in a social order in which a dozen individuals weigh more in the scale of importance than the other hundreds of millions forming a nation, and where is sanity in a system of publicity in which these hundreds of millions are strictly debarred from entry into this exclusive province, in which only the celebrities in politics, learning, wealth, commerce, art or athletics or notables in crime, deception, murder, rape, plunder or other villainies are allowed free access every moment to appease a self-created morbid hunger for excitement, inimical to the health of the brain? Do we ever remind ourselves that we are not exposing a piece of processed leather to the sun, rain and storm of the psychological weather around us, but the most sensitive, the most tender and the most delicate fabric in our mortal frame?

How does it happen that in a world nourished on the Bible, Quran, the Dhammapada and the Gita, all of them stressing the merits of humility, compassion, love of truth, temperance, austerity and fellow-feeling, that those who are the very embodiment of these virtues among the teeming crowds, gentle and modest, live and die in oblivion, their sterling worth, their acts of charity, nobility of character, sacrifice and courage never becoming known to serve as examples for the rest. On the contrary, the assassins or would-be assassins of presidents, prime ministers, popes or other dignitaries, heads of dacoits and gangster chiefs, the terrorist leaders and the smuggler-kings, the incurable rapists and the master-crooks, receive such glaring publicity that their evil faces and horrid acts bore into the memory and press upon the imagination of the masses, repeated again and again, until they erode the instinctive abhorrence felt and the aversion aroused against such abnormal creatures and their loathsome deeds.

The race is paying heavily for the commercialization of the news industry! Constant exposure to exciting and sensational events, dreadful incidents and ghastly scenes, stories of grisly crime and accounts of murder, plunder, terrorism, hijacking, shoot-outs and the rest, has a traumatic effect on the neurons of the brain, especially in the child and the adolescent. There can be no greater error than to suppose that the brain is immune to contagion and the contamination which affect the other organs and tissues of the body. On the contrary, considering the extremely delicate nature of the fabric of which it is made, a much greater degree of susceptibility is to be expected. Any act or occurrence alarming, shocking or abhorrent to the mind partakes in its nature of something which is inimical or lethal to human existence. Constant exposure to that which is uncongenial, dangerous or fatal to our survival, whether in actual encounter or in the form of news, is repugnant to and acts as poison on the brain, itself the ever-alert watchman and custodian of life.

No one can deny that our brain is, in some way, intimately connected with the expression of thought. How can it be possible then, that high excitement, acute suspense, explosive anger, overpowering shock, venomous hate, extreme horror or intense revulsion caused by screaming newspaper accounts, radio broadcasts and lurid television shows, cannot but adversely affect the neurons, creating lesions in the extremely fragile material, which we neither perceive nor can cure. It must never be forgotten that what is disquieting, distracting or revolting for the mind is disturbing and repellant for the grey-matter too.

The parental emphasis on good behavior and probity, coupled with scriptural injunctions in the case of religious-minded families, and what is seen daily with the eyes or heard with the ears, creates a conflict in the mind of the child which is reflected in the brain-matter. The scholars cannot perceive this growing shadow on the brain any more than they can observe the play of thought. The effect is not instantaneously perceptible but, as in other degenerative processes, may take decades or even generations to come to the surface. The damage, already done to the delicate texture of the cerebral cortex, especially among the advanced nations, by this complete disregard of hygiene of the brain, unless remedied at once, will increase in proportion as years roll by, until all the fire still burning in the virile stocks of today is extinguished, as happened irrevocably to the civilizations of the past, including those of Greece and Rome.

Another adverse effect of the present system is that it blunts the sensibility of the brain and its power of quick deterrant response to evil, essential for the safety and survival of the individual. The almost daily or oft-repeated appearance of the elite among politicians, administrators, traders, industrialists and the like, imprints their image on the public mind so firmly that, even when the malpractices, misdeeds, corruption or other faults of some among them come to light, they still continue to figure in the imaginations of the people, ready to stage a come-back again at a suitable opportunity. This is especially true of politicians, whose names or faces, even after shameful exposures, continue to haunt the mind and attract the attention of readers or television viewers on account of the strong imprint on the brain.

I have touched this topic, in passing, to bring into relief but one of the grave consequences resulting from the current woeful lack of knowledge about the brain. There are many others that would be discussed in future volumes. By a dispensation of Providence, the seat of our life, namely the brain, is so sensitive to the environment, so perceptive of the ills in a society and so acutely conscious of the wrongs and inequities done, at this present stage of evolution, that a sweeping change must occur in every sphere of human life to keep it healthy and sound. The instinctive rebellious attitude of young, resilient minds against the inequitable norms of present-day societies is the outcome of this ferment in the brain.

It can be safely asserted that the present crisis, the race for armaments, the deployment of nuclear weapons, the wars, bloody coups and violent uprisings, a slur on the race at the present height of culture, provide only a sample of the deterioration that has already set in the cerebral cortex of a section among the dominant brains. The insensitivity to the horrors of a nuclear war is a clear symptom of abnormality reminiscent of the war-frenzy of berserk Tartar hordes. The decay will continue unless the milieu is changed. Knowing full well what a delicate balance of the environment and what a marvellous adjustment of the elemental forces of nature were necessary for the nurture of life, and the appearance of man on this planet, can we doubt the obvious conclusion that the same delicate balance and the same marvellous adjustment is needed in the human society also to provide a salubrious milieu for her rise to a still higher performance of the brain. There are many who talk of evolution, mindless of the host of problems and the endless chain of intricate issues that follow in its wake.

Mystics in the illuminative state beget a conviction that they are in rapport with the source of all knowledge or that knowledge of the mysteries have been revealed to them. Some of them, as for instance Jacob Boehme and Ignatious Loyola, have clearly expressed this feeling. This is also the case with Bucke. Others, too, have given direct or indirect expression to this idea in their works. Viewed in the context of this aspect of mystical ecstasy, the final and even the mandatory character of the gospels of various faiths is not hard to understand. Abstract thinking and reasoning, a distinctive feature of the human plane of consciousness, is absent in that of animals. On this analogy, what should we expect when the human plane is transcended? The answer is supra-rational knowledge of the kind which the founders of revealed faiths and even some mystics say was communicated to them. The very style and wording of the scriptures of current faiths seem to be instinct with the idea that the contents were received in a direct communication from an infallible Source of all knowledge or God.

This peculiar feature of the gospels is not surprising for the reason that the extension of consciousness signifies extension of knowledge and enhancement of intelligence. To the subject of the experience, it appears as if he is immersed in one vast ocean of super-human knowledge and intelligence combined and has nothing more to learn. The idea continues to persist even when the ecstasy is over. Probably, due to the limitation of the brain in some cases, the experience ends with a subjective feeling only, and no real addition to the knowledge of the mundane or super-mundane world filters down into the normal consciousness of the subject. In other cases, there is a definite gain in knowledge and high refinement in the power of expression. The two often assume the form of inspired verse and prose, exclusively applied to the Transcendental. As a harvest of these newly acquired gifts, we have a large store of beautiful and inspiring gems of literature, left as a legacy by great mystics, both in the East and the West, expressive of what they braved and endured on the path, the glorious prize they won, and what it symbolizes for the world. These masterpieces survive intact today, hundreds and even thousands of years after they were penned.

One of the main distinguishing features of genuine transcen-dental experience is that it must bequeath to one who has it a momento of the visit to the Empyrean world. Otherwise, how can one differentiate between a dream, a delusion or a real ascent to the abode of gods? One who has arrived at the Shrine of Life must bring back a token to show that the pilgrimage was done. The scriptures of various faiths and the accounts of their ascent, left behind by many of the great mystics, are all eloquent testimonials to the visit paid. The pilgrimage must climax in an artistic crea-tion or supra-rational knowledge of some kind. It is chiefly through this sign that the prophets and oracles of yore were accepted by their contemporaries. It is the one unmistakable token by which they can be recognized even now.

It is not by the mere avowal of a visionary that his alleged encounter with God or Cosmic Intelligence can be accepted as a genuine transcendental experience, but by the impact it has on his life and the knowledge vouchsafed for communication to the world. The knowledge must not be borrowed or stale or false or obscure, incapable of withstanding the scrutiny of contemporaries or the test of time. It must be original and lucid, couched in a language appropriate to the lofty theme, providing wholesome food for the hungry souls waiting to hear more and more about this super-earthly excursion to the region beyond. The voyage might have been rough, the weather stormy, the ocean tempestuous and the vessel ploughing its way through, rickety and frail, but once arrived at the port, all the trials are forgotten, all the sorrows are overcome, all the sufferings cease in the enchanting melody and ravishing beauty of the new haven of joy, where the Soul, exhausted by the struggle for existence, and scorched by the fever of the world, finds rest and repose at last.

Anyone who claims to have transcended the limits of human intelligence, however brief the interlude might have been, must produce evidence in support to affix the seal of confirmation on the statement that the adventurous voyage was done, the other shore reached and, on the way back, a few grains of the golden soil were picked up, as a souvenir, to bring home on one's return to his native soil. When we expect anyone who lands on the moon to bring back a few handfuls of the lunar soil or one who visits a far away shrine to show us some relic of the holy place, should we not ask one who claims to have visited the Kingdom of Heaven what rare treasure he picked up there and what gem of wisdom he brought back to share with the world?

How can I claim to have made this voyage and sailed to the wondrous land beyond the frontiers of mind until I show a proof to convince the world that I have really been there? What can I say to those who ask me for an account of my travels and the knick-knacks that I gathered in that land of dreams? For this reason, it behooves me to narrate my experiences as best I can, and to show the souvenirs I collected in the course of the voyage to the idyllic Shore. I cannot say that I made a rich haul. The mediocrity of my natural mental endowment, the poverty of knowledge and the

gruelling ordeals I had to face throughout on account of my
ignorance of the path, make my collection extremely meagre,
but sufficient to demonstrate the truth of what I say. What wealth
of knowledge the future voyagers shall bring in the days ahead,
to enrich the race with spiritual treasures, is beyond conception
at present.

The most precious relic I was allowed to pick up in the divine
territory relates to a momentous secret of the brain, which is still
hidden from the human world. I do not say this knowledge is a
part of a supernatural revelation or supernatural encounter. But
it formed a part of my experience and slowly dawned on me, not
as the harvest of my own intellectual effort, but as the fruit of the
changes I underwent during the course of my extraordinary pilgrimage. I do not claim that the secret revealed has made me a
specialist in phrenology or in the neurology of the brain or a
wizard with a cabbalistic knowledge of this organ. What I have
learned is that the human encephalon already has embedded in it
the scroll of man's future destiny, as also the key to his rise to
another dimension of consciousness where, for the first time,
light begins to dawn on his own mystery.

Apart from the bewildering complexity of its formation and
the incredible range of its activities, the world has still no awareness of the real marvel of the brain. We never realize, when looking at the brow of a fellow being, that inside the osseous dome the
whole universe is contained in but one particle of a divine substance, smaller than a grain of salt, smaller even than the smallest
fragment that we can see. It is not to the pineal or the pituitary
gland that I refer; it is not to any part of the brain material, but the
wonder which builds it in the womb and uses it as its instrument to
enact the drama of life in every individual. The 'wonder' which,
though all-knowing and all-seeing, contrives its own imprison-
ment in a house of clay, witnesses its own growth from childhood
to old age, participating in a long chain of experiences, some plea-
sant and some painful, all originating from the wonder-stuff of
which it is itself composed.

We never see the power animating the brain; never come

across the mysterious Source of our life; never glimpse the Guardian Angel that wakes us up every morning, rested and refreshed, to attend to our daily chores with our limbs and organs, kept in readiness to do our bidding by the same Angel, in a manner unperceived by us. We never know that this Wonder in the brain knows all that is past, all that is to come, all that happens in every part of the universe, on the suns and planets, on the beds of the oceans or in the interior of the earth. Its power is unlimited, its knowledge infallible, its memory unfailing, its imagination all-creative and its will all-powerful, and yet it is the helpless infant, the crippled soldier and the lame beggar bent low with age.

I am not talking of the Creator, I am not alluding to God, I do not refer to any supernatural Being when I describe the attributes of this marvel in the brain. What I am trying to communicate is something different, something which I experienced and verified, something which it is necessary for mankind to know to be out of the prisons in science, philosophy and even religion in which she has confined herself. This something is not a stranger to the universe in which we live; something exotic or foreign to it, but another mighty element of creation in the same way as mind and matter, or that from which they both emerge, are its elements and have been accepted as such from immemorial times. The creation round us does not consist of mind and matter alone, or only as one of them as the materialists or their opponents, the idealists, contend, but of layer after layer, element after element, plane after plane of, for us, inconceivable energies and forces, stuffs and substances, that are as dissimilar to the materials and forces among which we live as sky is from the earth, ether from a rock or light from gloom.

This is the reason why I am turning out book after book to apprise the world that creation does not consist of what we call spirit and matter alone, that the universe we perceive is but one out of myriads running parallel to each other, sometimes occupying the same space, or what we know as space, formed of diverse, what we name material components, each imperceptible to the other, each with its own layout, its own expanse, boundaries, plan, its own dwellers, order, values, rules and laws. We have travelled very far from the geocentric viewpoint of our distant ancestors in our assessment of the material universe. But in our assessment of the spiritual kingdom we are still where we were thousands of years ago. On the corporeal side, we live in a body which, in turn, dwells in a house. The house is located in a village or town which, in turn, forms the part of a country, spread over a large or small portion of our planet. The earth, in its turn, forms a part of the solar system and the solar system of a galaxy.

We do not regard the earth now as the center or the hub of creation, but as a minor planet in a solar system among billions in our galaxy alone, and billions upon billions in other galaxies, already formed, and billions more in those still in the state of formation in other parts of the universe. But, so far as our psychic side is concerned, we still believe that the same intelligence or maybe some more evolved form of it, as we possess, is spread all over the cosmos. In other words, we project on a creation of such a staggering magnitude, of such varied forms, dimensions and durations, one uniform pattern of consciousness modelled, more or less, on the human type, even in extra-terrestrial or extra-galactic forms of life without enlarging in the least our concept about the world of mind and its cosmic manifestations, as we have done in the case of the material world. Would it not be more realistic to imagine the same variegation and the same gradation of consciousness in its other planetary and galactic manifestations, as we perceive in the material content of the Cosmos?

This is a multi-faced, multi-dimensional and multi-tudinous universe. Humanity lives and dies in but one out of innumerable planes of consciousness that exist in it. Her sensory equipment is only for this one particular plane of existence. The same is true of her mind. She can no more perceive the other planes or their inhabitants than a blind eye can see the colors of a rainbow. The material world with its nebulae, galactic systems, stars, planets and moons is but a gross replica of the unbounded spiritual universe. There are, as it were, psychic nebulae, galactic systems, suns, planets and moons with their inhabitants, separated from each other by insuperable barriers, not of time and space, but varied instruments of sensory perception. The dwellers in each plane, like the dwellers on earth, have their own sensory equipment, designed for the particular plane of the multi-dimensional universe in which they live. Our dream experience, the latest concepts of physics, the inexplicable psychic phenomena, the widespread ancient belief in devas, angels, fairies, gnomes, jinn, demons and the like, archaic legends, mythologies and folktales, faith in ascended Masters and living adepts, as also the experiences of mystics, all point in the same direction.

The Creator is far, far away. The Lord of this infinite creation, though everywhere, is yet further away than the last limit, if any, of the universe. There are countless planes of consciousness and countless barriers of the sensory walls to be crossed before He can be reached. The Quest will never end as long as humanity is allowed to stay on earth. She might, with the knowledge gained of subtle forces of creation, in the foreseeable future migrate from planet to planet in her physical body, and rise to plane after plane of transcendental consciousness, with the continued evolution of her brain. What skies will open before her, what horizons melt, what barriers she would overcome, what tempests brace, what sights would meet her eyes, what wonders she would see shall be the saga of the future, packed with romance, adventure, transport and delight, before which all the sagas of the past would fall into shade.

The panorama of life on the earth, from the primary forms to the towering intellect of man, provides a specimen to show that similar gradations might be existing in other planes or other parts of the cosmos. Our human awareness, with all its wealth of intelligence, compared to the conscient giants inhabiting those other planes, might be corresponding only to the feeble glimmer of sentience in the lower forms of terrestrial life. In the other planes, intelligence, rising higher and higher in power and volume, might have reached those unimaginable proportions which we associate with gods.

How long can we stick to the homocentric idea that the human soul, by dint of hard spiritual disciplines, can take a sudden leap to be one with the Almighty, or, in other words, with one bound attain to omnipotence and wisdom absolute, as many among the illuminati aver can be the case? Would it not be more sensible to assume that earth is not the only amphitheater for man to stage the drama of his life, but that there are countless others, more spacious and more magnificent than that of this planet, where attired in other costumes, more ethereal than the one he wears now, he is destined to play far superior roles, in front of other audiences belonging to the same planetary species as he?

After witnessing the amazing progress made by mankind during the last two centuries and the possibilities of inter-planetary travel opened by technology, can we still continue to harbor the same out-of-date geocentric idea that humanity is forever condemned to internment in a body of earthy clay, restricting her peregrinations only to different parts of the earth or, at the most, to planets of the solar system, where her organic frame can survive the rigor of the new environment? Would it not be wiser to assume that there can also be a similar spurt in the spiritual progress of the race, with the knowledge of a momentous secret of life, as happened on the physical plane with the discovery of certain, till lately, unknown laws of matter, and that the two combined may lead to a revolution that would make her as great an adept in the knowledge of the subtler forces of nature as she is of the grosser ones?

Mystical experience, understood in its true color as the entry into another dimension of consciousness, presents a new vision of human destiny. Man is not born to starve, emasculate or mortify himself, or to shun the world, as a precondition to court the favor of the Lord, until the boon is granted in a state of ecstasy, and then to disappear from the arena of his activity on the earth like a rabbit in its hole. Such a view of creation would be an affront to a Cosmic Intelligence. It would reduce the colossal drama of existence to a puppet show in which the puppets dance round the Master the whole time and, in the last act, chant his praises and kiss the ground under his feet, before the curtain drops. Can such

a gross exhibition of vanity and self-love befit the paragon of all
that is noble, true and pure in creation? Can such a selfish father
prove a healthy example for the progeny?

In the light of our present-day knowledge of the Cosmos, can
we impute such a lack of feeling to the Maker, that He would pres-
cribe such a fatuous climax to mark the end of a long-drawn,
agonizing climb, covering millions of years, every inch of which is
drenched with blood and tears? Or, at the end of a hazardous
aeonean adventure, as soon as the going becomes easier, and the
participants find a little leisure to look around and refresh themselves, force them to desist on pain of eternal damnation and
ceaseless torment in the other world? Can this be the plan of a
compassionate God, to subject his creatures to the severest
ordeals in a savage setting until they attain the degree of intelligence to reshape the harsh environment to their choice, and then
to expect them to renounce the well-earned rest and restart
another cycle of fasts, self-denials, privations, laments, prayers
and tears to the exclusion of every other heart-warming, genial
effort, in order to express their love and devotion for Him?

No, such an interpretation of mystical experience cannot be
correct. Divine Intelligence cannot be guilty of such incongruities
in her creations. The error lies in projecting our own frailties on
the divine Architect. There must be a purpose in man's appearance on earth. The agony of birth, the discomforts of teething,
measles, whooping cough and other ailments of childhood mark
but the beginning of the long, adventurous life of a human being.
The same must be true of the human race. The child's dreams of
supermen, invincible heroes, angels, fairies, other-worldly beings,
wonder-creations and the like, might be more true of the future
man than what the learned know or can forecast about him today.
It cannot be without purpose that nature has placed all the
resources of an entire planet, with the prodigious animal, plant
and mineral wealth completely at the pleasure of this intellectual
giant whose height of ambition outsoars the stars.

Without awareness of the other planes of creation, humanity
will continue to regard the prison house erected around her by

the brain as her permanent dwelling place, designed by nature in which she is forever fore-doomed to live. Migration to other planets in the solar system, even if possible, will not demolish the sensory prison walls. Her elite will continue to devote all their time and energy to make the lock-house as comfortable as possible for the entire stock and the progeny. One after the other they will look around it, explore it, try to know its formation and measure its extent, as they are doing now. Denied an eschatological outlet, the race is likely to become more and more ease-loving, with the products of technology, and come more and more into the grip of luxury, sensuality and indolence.

Without a pull from above, perhaps in no more than a century, the novelty of the mechanical wonders our intellect has devised will wear away, and people will start to feel as bored, as frustrated and as dissatisfied with their lot as they had ever felt before. When this happens and the glamor of today's achievements has faded, the deep-rooted urge to break away from the sensory prison will grip their imagination and sour their life of ease once again. This has even started to happen now. Those who believe that by surfeit, luxurious lifestyles and multiplications of needs, man will live a happy and contented life on earth are gravely mistaken. He will spurn it all and revert to pastoral occupations and spartan ways of life, if that helps him more to liberate himself. The divine in him will never allow this wonder-child of Heaven to barter his kingdom-to-come for the trinkets of the earth.

EPILOGUE

Before the preordained glorious consummation of her aeon-ean pilgrimage, humanity must know more about her divine origin, the imperishable Splendor within, the fragile temple of clay it dwells in, and the life she must lead to fulfil her destiny. By a strange quirk of fate, the phenomenal progress she made during the last few centuries in gaining mastery over the forces of nature, has made her even poorer in the knowledge about her self. But one false step taken by the aristocracy of her intellect in relegating the mind to a secondary position as compared to the body—a palpable oversight—is at the bottom of the present crisis, which needs a counter-revolution in thought to defuse it. Her amazing achievements—abundance, wealth, advancement of learning, conquest over distance, time, disease and famine, unprecedented luxury, comfort and easements, wonders of space travel, marvels of surgery, the glamor and romance of an exciting and delightful life and the prospect of greater triumphs in future—all combined, cannot undo the consequences of the over-sight. If the mistake is not rectified, she would meet the same fate as she did over and over again in the vanished civilizations of the past.

The signs of this deterioration are visible even now. Only a keener sight and wider knowledge is needed to discern them. This sight and this knowledge is the perogative of sober minds that have gained the ability to look beyond the gaudy trappings of a passing show. The current perverse way of thinking that allots the first position to what is perishable and false, and the last to what is enduring and true is slowly cutting at the roots of the society. The great kingdoms and the ascendant nations of the past thought and behaved in the same way after attaining to lofty heights of culture and prosperity, only a few steps lower than ours. They fell because, at a certain point of their ascent, they did not know how to proceed further and came rolling down the slope never to rise again. The modern civilization is threatened in the same way on account of the same lack of knowledge of the path. The downward slide has already begun and, because of the greater height gained, the speed of the descent is more precipitate than ever was the case before!

I hope I shall not be misunderstood if I make bold to say that the guiding lights of the race have lost the way, deceived by the luxuriant bloom of their intellect and the rank profusion of their creations. They fail to see, misled by the exuberance of the summer crop, that the icy chill of winter is ready to descend on the gorgeous scene. Why? Because, as the result of over-confidence in our mental endowment, based on an exaggerated picture of its capability, we are devoting by far more attention to the superfluous than the essential, to the branches than to the root in the false belief that our knowledge is comprehensive and correct. Let me take a single example. No one can deny that nature—blind and unintelligent, as we assume her to be—has taken extraordinary pains in designing and fashioning the head of the human body in order to protect from harm its extremely fragile occupant—the brain—a rare masterpiece of super-human craftsmanship, still a sealed book to the erudite.

Layer after layer of protective sheaths, some tough and some of downy softness, interpose between the rough skull and the body of the delicate tenant, as a lining to its hard interior, to serve as a velvety cushion for the extremely tender inmate within. The skull itself is a thick, bony structure, dome-shaped for extra strength, covered with a wooly padding of hair to protect it from blows, knocks, strokes, bumps, heat, cold, radiation and the like. Apart from this triple line of defense, the cerebro-spinal fluid fills every fissure, cavity, nook and corner of the brain to act as a stress, jerk, jolt and shock absorber of incredible potency. The blood supply is so skillfully arranged that the chances of a failure are extremely curtailed. Apart from all this, there are ingenious devices in the sensory organs, directly linked to the brain, to prevent harm or pollution from coming in through them. There is no other organ of the body, including the precious heart and the priceless eyes, so well enclosed and protected against a rough environment and the possibility of injury as in this seat of life.

At the time of birth, the head comes out first, protected by a marvellous fluidic cushion to ensure safety for this extremely delicate organ, always to be handled with tender care. But with this example of the extraordinary precautions taken by Nature before our eyes, how do most of us more understanding and far better informed than before, behave with this soveriegn part of our mortal frame? Does it command priority in our daily roster of tasks and more attention than to other parts of the body? To be honest it does not. Far from that, it does not even figure in our daily thoughts at all. To enhance our beauty, charm, symmetry or strength do we not pay ten times more attention to the face, body and limbs than to the head? Are not beauty parlors, gymnasiums, massage salons, face-lifting clinics, swimming pools, Turkish and sauna baths, sports fields, golf courses, tennis courts, race tracks and the like, galore everywhere to attest the attention we pay to and the fondness we have for the other parts of our organic frame. Does the care of the head figure anywhere in these numerous departments of body care?

How we repay the tender care of nature and treat this holy shrine of the soul is obvious from our complete lack of interest in and absence of regard for this master of our body whom she is so anxious to protect. Do not the pugilists make of it the first target for their smashing fists, the wrestlers for their crushing holds, the enthusiasts of self-defense a battering ram to floor their opponents, sturdy footballers a bat to hit back a streaking ball, the Asans—zealots a stool to support their inverted trunk and legs in the air, keen swimmers a wedge to cleave the water with when diving from giddy heights, and so on. When closely examined, there surely will be found many other instances of this abuse.

Do not even fond parents make this precious part of their child or its component, the face, their first choice for a box or a slap as a corrective for misbehavior, gentle ladies, when violent, their favorite site for scratching with nails or tearing out each other's hair; ardent lovers, when excited, the ideal place to pinch hard and bite the beloved, children, in fun, their butt to squeeze tightly under the elbow, and belabor with shoes, satchels or fists and mature grownups, to vent their rage, their chosen spot to hit with stones, beat with sticks, rain shattering blows on, shake violently by the throat or dash against a nearby wall of solid brick or stone? Has anyone, I ask, raised his voice against this desecration of the shrine of life, the most precious and the most tender organ in our body which nature takes endless pains to guard?

Do we not expose this full-blown, exquisite flower of thought, unprotected to blistering heat and biting cold for sheer bravado, to jolts, jerks and knocks for fun and frivolity, to dizzy speed and giddy sport for amusement, to grinding labor and killing work for gain or fame, to sleepless nights and hectic days for nocturnal revel and even-tide sickly pleasure, without ever reminding ourselves that, as in the case of our other organs and limbs—heart, lungs, stomach, arms and legs—the resources of the brain cannot be unlimited and that there must be a border beyond which it is not safe to proceed.

Apart from all these excesses, do we not in our self-escalated battle of life and frantic search for a front seat make this invaluable organ a helpless tool for our selfish designs, subjecting it to tension and distraction in pursuit of over-ambitious dreams, to ceaseless worry and anxiety as the fruit of acute rivalry and competition or to fear and fright by fostering hate and enmity? On top of these do we not expose it needlessly to rapid change of emotions—excitement, shock, terror, revulsion, suspense and the rest by senile infatuation with the sensation-loving news media, and immoderate passion for thrilling novels, exciting fiction, horror stories or bizarre narratives perused endlessly at all hours? Lastly, besides all this, do we not repeatedly subject it to angry outbursts and emotional storms, so furious they leave even the tough body sick and exhausted, what to say of the hypersensitive cerebral lobes?

Above all, do not most of us sell this priceless treasure dirt cheap to its sworn enemies—bemusing drugs, befuddling wine and begriming tobacco—beyond a certain limit, all three sure poisons for the cerebro-spinal Tree of Life? Heaven alone knows to what monstrous degree we are out to undo with our own hands the master-work which it took patient nature millions of years to complete for the simple reason that, even at her present height of culture, mankind is still a stranger to her own brain?

The fanatics who believe that human beings can carry on with impunity in any environment or dwell safely on man-built satellites orbiting the earth, or that families can be sent in rockets designed for exploration of distant planets, needing a life-time to reach, and then return to earth in the second or third generation, are living in a paradise of fools. The first internal study of the living brain will make the empiricists involved reel back in awed silence and surprise, for nature has concentrated all her ingenuity in this organic masterpiece. It is well to remember that there exists every device and every artifice in the brain to prevent the human race by her exuberant intellect from swerving even an inch from the path aligned for her. She shall either follow it or extinguish herself. This is the reason why the victorious empires of the past, often at the zenith of their glory, came tumbling down to earth to roll in dust for centuries, in the grip of delusive ideas of greatness, vain-glorious customs, unhealthy habits and unwholesome appetites. Humanity might be able to achieve anything by her matchless wit: flout the physical laws of nature, dry up oceans, inundate deserts, level mountains or make her home in the skies, but she never will be able to by-pass the brain to escape her destiny.

Every word that I write is to be treated as a solemn affirmation of one who, by a strange dispensation of Providence, was led to an internal observation of his own brain, day and night, for a period of nearly forty-five years. The knowledge gathered, rudimentary and imperfect at this stage, will take volumes to fill. It is this hidden knowledge of the fountain-head of our life which is the aim of my life to bring to light. All that I write is not to be treated as a revelation in the usually accepted sense of the term, nor as a communication from a supernatural source, but as the carefully observed data of a normal human being—initially more of an agnostic than a believer—who has been irresistibly led to the conclusions expressed after he had exhausted every explanation he could think of to throw light on the occurrences in any other way.

Even so, the observations made and the conclusions drawn are not to be accepted unless confirmed by a series of experiments done by other servants of humanity who believe that the tenets expounded have a degree of plausibility, entitling the phenomenon to further investigation in order to arrive at the truth. Nothing would grant me greater happiness than to see the start of a massive wave of interest in the internal exploration of the cerebral Temple and the Divine Light within, that has been the aim of every spiritual and occult discipline ever practised on the earth. It is my prayer that, considering the magnitude of the phenomenon that I am relating and its paramount importance for the race, the subject may not be a topic of frivolous controversy over trifles, but an issue for sober reflection and fruitful discussion, demanding a healthy exercise of the intellect on either side. From those who for whatever reason turn up their nose in contempt at the avowals made, I humbly implore patience, reminding them of the truth that, "there are more things in heaven and earth than we can ever know of."

It is good to remember that the object under discussion is the matchless asset and the very spring of life in every human being. But from all that is happening, it is clear that the people are not really conscious of the savior they carry in their head. For instance, how many of us reflect on the fact that every time we fall into the oblivion of sleep at night, we entrust ourselves without knowing it into the hands of a Guardian Angel who looks into every nook and corner of our reclining figure and with a gentle, feather touch makes order where a jumble has been caused by our hectic or aggressive activity during the day?

When awake in the morning, refreshed and calmed, cured of a mental fever or a bodily ailment by a restful sleep, how many of us send thanks to Providence for the priceless boon of the heavenly nurse who puts us to bed when, like naughty children, we have bruised ourselves in careless frolic and reckless sport, torn our dress with the brambles and thorns of vice, wickedness, excess or violence, or soiled our face and hands with the dirt of impure, crooked, spiteful, vindictive or treacherous thought or act and wakes us up after healing the cuts, repairing the rents and washing clean the stains to make us presentable once again. How many of the wealthiest, the most learned and the mightiest of the earth ever realize that, after retiring to bed at night, now like other humble creatures no more inflated by their greatness, they rise in the morning the same as they had gone to sleep, to continue the thread of their life of affluence, academic honor or high command, only because the divine healer had been at work in their brain while they were lost to themselves and their applauding world.

Our ceaseless activity of thought and endless play of emotions, from the tenderest to the most violent, make an ever-present process of repair an essential requirement of our cranial machine. The amount of bio-energy used in this continuous work of renewal and restoration depends on the extent of the wear and tear or the impairment caused. A balanced life of equanimity, patience and forbearance makes the process of repair less exacting, with less expenditure of the precious organic fuels sustaining life. With every improvement in the mental calibre of a population, there must come about a corresponding improvement in the repair mechanism, as in the mode of life to prevent excessive consumption of the vital essences. For this reason, at every stage of the mental or cultural progress of a people, concordance must prevail between the advancing intellect and the way of life of the multitudes. If this does not happen, the canker of decay invades the mass.

It might be argued that over-occupation with the brain and over-attention to its care can become an obsession bound to curtail one's freedom and hamper the performance of other duties. To say the least, this is an imaginary fear. Our primitive ancestors walked barefoot over stones and thorns, squatted on bare earth, ate with unclean hands and took no notice of bodily hygiene at all. We have now learned to take good care of our feet, use fine socks and shoes, take a morning bath, pare our nails at intervals and wash our hands several times a day. This daily routine, the fruit of our culture, has not become an obsession nor does it interfere in any way with our normal schedule of work. On the other hand, it saves us from dirt and infection and makes us feel more composed and refreshed in attending to our duties during the day. But apart from using a headcover by day and a pillow at night, in contrast to our distant forbear who went bare-headed (except in the glacial periods) and stretched his uncovered body on the ground at night, we have not advanced much in our treatment of the encephalon, save giving it a wash and occasional trimming or cropping of the hair.

Beyond that we have hardly made any progress compared to the care we lavish on the other parts of the body, exposed to view or used for movement and manual work. On the contrary, at least in one direction, we are even more careless than our savage ancestor. Denied the spectacle of alluring beauty and scintillating lights at night and less voluptuous in thought, from scanty food and hard exertion during the day, he usually followed the natural hours of sleep, allowing good rest to his growing brain. The result was that he progressed slowly, until the leisure and sensuous allurements of civilized life, leading to indolence, intemperance, abuse, excess, intoxication, late hours, unhealthy excitement, vice and venality, acting on the delicate organ—most precious and now most abused by him—brought every civilization he erected irretrievably to the earth. The rationalists believe that the elements and forces of nature surrounding us are dead; that the wind blows and the earth rotates in concordance with inviolable physical laws, and that man is the monarch of all that he surveys as there is no sign or evidence to prove the existence of a divine power or a Master-Mind behind the vast creation known to us. They argue in this vein because they have little knowledge of the very source from which this thinking comes. If the ancient physicians had been as knowledgeable in the distempers of the brain as they were in the diseases of the body, the history of mankind would have been radically different and the nations that once rose to the pinnacle of power would never have lost their supremacy. Similarly, were the erudite of today as highly versed in the knowledge of this organ as they are in the other parts of the human frame, the race would not be facing a serious threat to her life at this time. That is the reason why the foremost nations of our day, commanding the richest and most fertile intellectual talent the earth has ever seen, display the same symptoms and are poised for the same fall.

The rise and fall of empires, kingdoms, royal dynasties, princely houses, aristocracies and wealthy families presents a most instructive phenomenon of history. The erudite, even when professing belief in God, seldom envision the existence of a divine law ruling the fate of human-kind. For many of the believers God is a figure-head who lets His creatures manage their affairs as they like. It is hard to imagine for a dry intellect that every quantum leap of an atomic particle, every descent of a raindrop and every fall of a leaf happens under command. We are encompassed by an Intelligence beyond the widest flight of human thought. The recent studies of the marvellous code embedded in a gene should have proved sufficient to humble our pride, but it has had a contrary effect and made many of us proud of our own ability in discovering it. We seldom imagine, when face to face with a wonder of creation, that the Intelligence behind it surpasses our understanding a million times more than we surpass the understanding of a mole.

Our own brain marks the frontier where the human wit must come to a halt. From it the territory forbidden to the intellect begins. This is the place of confluence where the divine and the mundane meet. The most minute scrutiny of the organ carried on for ages would only show the corporeal. The cerebral chamber must be illuminated from within to light up for us the otherwise invisible planes of creation to which our mind and spirit belong. Inner Light has been a common feature of all genuine mystical experiences, irrespective of the place and the period of time. The appearance of this splendour marks the opening of a new center of perception in the brain, vital for the knowledge of supersensory worlds. With this endowment, a new chapter in the life of an individual is opened, a new heroic adventure and a new illuminating study begin.

There was a time when human beings viewed the epidemics of smallpox, plague or cholera as the work of evil spirits or as a visitation from heaven against which no human effort could prevail. Our attitude of mind towards the ascension and decline of ancient kingdoms and of the moral deterioration occurring before our eyes is, more or less, the same. Humanity is in grave jeopardy because she faces a deplorable lack of expert advisers on the organ of her thought. Looking at specialists and experts in every sphere of human activity, interest or need, from the care of feet to the exploration of space, or from the culture of bees to the nuclear Armageddon, it is heart-rending to find a gaping void where the space should have been most crowded to keep the race well posted about the state of health and efficiency of the sole arbiter of her destiny, the one very delicate instrument of her life, progress, happiness and survival on which all her other interests depend, that is, her brain!

The ideal will be realized when, in the years to come, expert knowledge of the incorporeal and the corporeal constituents of the human encephalon is combined in the same specialist. This combination of the sage and the scientist would be the harbinger of a Golden Age for humanity. Intuition and reason must walk hand in hand to prepare the race for her existence in both the sensory and super-sensory worlds. No one can be more surprised than I am at the unbelievable results that followed my staggering experience in December, 1937. Had I heard the same story from the lips of another before I underwent the experience myself, I would have found it hard to believe the narrator, even if I knew that he was a strict adherent of truth. It is, therefore, no shock to me when I fail to enlist belief from those who hear or read my narrative.

I never ceased to be a self-critic, even after my entry to the lustrous plane which forms the wonder-gallery of my life. Repeatedly I ask myself, as I would ask a stranger: how does it happen that an obscure creature, so poor in academic attainments, so unimpressive among the glittering assemblies of the earth, and so acutely conscious of his insignificance in so vast an amphitheater, should push himself forward at this particular time to call attention to a serious omission in the knowledge of the learned about an important subject of utmost urgency for the race. But knowing how inscrutable are the ways of Providence, I content myself with the answer that I should accept it as my destiny and do all that I can to perform the duty that now devolves on me with truth, honesty and proper care, until the Light that brought the summons discards the body, which is now executing it, to mingle with the splendor wherein she dwells, letting the dress of clay return to the earth wherefrom it came.

To divert attention towards a new subject of study is a hard task to achieve. In this case, it is more so as it involves a departure from the current methods employed for the study of mind. Secondly, the subject itself is likely to be frowned upon as an archaic superstition paraded in disguise. The reason is that there are always only a few who reflect seriously on an entirely new concept or an unexpected line of thought and fewer still who can envision the future possibilities inherent in it. But there always are courageous men and women who, intuitively drawn to the new idea and convinced of its importance, dedicate their lives, their time, talent and resources to find out and disseminate the Truth. It is by the noble effort and heroic sacrifice of this rare class of benefactors that the race has progressed, so far, and shall continue to do so in the ages to come.

Gopi Krishna

October 5, 1982
Rajpur Road,
Dehra Dun, (U.P.)
India

ABOUT THE AUTHOR

Gopi Krishna was born in 1903 to parents of Kashmiri Brahmin extraction. His birthplace was a small village about twenty miles from the city of Srinagar, the summer capital of the Jammu and Kashmir State in northern India. He spent the first eleven years of his life growing up in this beautiful Himalayan valley.

In 1914, his family moved to the city of Lahore in the Punjab which, at that time, was a part of British India. Gopi Krishna passed the next nine years completing his public school education. Illness forced him to leave the torrid plains of the Punjab and he returned to the cooler climate of the Kashmir Valley. During the succeeding years, he secured a post in the Public Works Department of the state, married and raised a family.

In 1946 he founded a social organization and with the help of a few friends tried to bring about reforms in some of the outmoded customs of his people. Their goals included the abolition of the dowry system, which subjected the families of brides to severe and even ruinous financial obligations, and the strictures against the remarriage of widows. After a few years, Gopi Krishna was granted premature retirement from his position in the government and devoted himself almost exclusively to service work in the community.

In 1967, he published his first major book in India, *Kundalini — The Evolutionary Energy in Man.* Shortly thereafter it was published in Great Britain and the United States and has since appeared in eleven major languages. The book presented to the Western world for the first time a clear and concise autobiographical account of the phenomenon of the awakening of Kundalini, which he had experienced in 1937. This work, and the sixteen other published books by Gopi Krishna have generated a steadily growing interest in the subjects of consciousness and the evolution of the brain. He also travelled extensively in Europe and North America, energetically presenting his theories to scientists, scholars, researchers and others.

Gopi Krishna's experiences led him to hypothesize that there is a biological mechanism in the human body which is responsible for creativity, genius, psychic abilities, religious and mystical experiences, as well as aberrant mental states. He asserted that ignorance of the working of this evolutionary mechanism was the main reason for the present dangerous state of world affairs. He called for a full scientific investigation of his hypothesis and believed that such an objective analysis would uncover the secrets of human evolution. It is this knowledge, he believed, that would give mankind the means to progress in peace and harmony.

Gopi Krishna passed away in July 1984 of a severe lung infection and is survived by his wife, three children and grandchildren. The work that he began is currently being carried forward through the efforts of a number of affiliated foundations, organizations and individuals around the world.